RELIGION AND SEXUALITY

Sexuality Studies Series

This series focuses on original, provocative, scholarly research examining from a range of perspectives the complexity of human sexual practice, identity, community, and desire. Books in the series explore how sexuality interacts with other aspects of society, such as law, education, feminism, racial diversity, the family, policing, sport, government, religion, mass media, medicine, and employment. The series provides a broad public venue for nurturing debate, cultivating talent, and expanding knowledge of human sexual expression, past and present.

Other volumes in the series are:

Masculinities without Men? Female Masculinity in Twentieth-Century Fictions, by Jean Bobby Noble
Every Inch a Woman: Phallic Possession, Femininity, and the Text, by Carellin Brooks
Queer Youth in the Province of the "Severely Normal," by Gloria Filax
The Manly Modern: Masculinity in Postwar Canada, by Christopher Dummitt
Sexing the Teacher: School Sex Scandals and Queer Pedagogies, by Sheila L. Cavanagh
Undercurrents: Queer Culture and Postcolonial Hong Kong, by Helen Hok-Sze Leung
Sapphistries: A Global History of Love between Women, by Leila J. Rupp
The Canadian War on Queers: National Security as Sexual Regulation, by Gary Kinsman and Patrizia Gentile
Awfully Devoted Women: Lesbian Lives in Canada, 1900-65, by Cameron Duder
Judging Homosexuals: A History of Gay Persecution in Quebec and France, by Patrice Corriveau
Sex Work: Rethinking the Job, Respecting the Workers, by Colette Parent, Chris Bruckert, Patrice Corriveau, Maria Nengeh Mensah, and Louise Toupin
Selling Sex: Experience, Advocacy, and Research on Sex Work in Canada, edited by Emily van der Meulen, Elya M. Durisin, and Victoria Love
The Man Who Invented Gender: Engaging the Ideas of John Money, by Terry Goldie

RELIGION AND SEXUALITY

Diversity and the Limits of Tolerance

EDITED BY

**Pamela Dickey Young, Heather Shipley,
and Tracy J. Trothen**

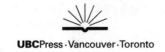

UBCPress · Vancouver · Toronto

© UBC Press 2015

All rights reserved. No part of this publication may be reproduced, stored in a retrieval system, or transmitted, in any form or by any means, without prior written permission of the publisher, or, in Canada, in the case of photocopying or other reprographic copying, a licence from Access Copyright, www.accesscopyright.ca.

23 22 21 20 19 18 17 16   5 4 3 2

Printed in Canada on FSC-certified ancient-forest-free paper (100% post-consumer recycled) that is processed chlorine- and acid-free.

Library and Archives Canada Cataloguing in Publication

Religion and sexuality : diversity and the limits of tolerance / edited by Pamela Dickey Young, Heather Shipley, and Tracy J. Trothen.

(Sexuality studies series)
Includes bibliographical references and index.
Issued in print and electronic formats.

ISBN 978-0-7748-2869-7 (bound). – ISBN 978-0-7748-2870-3 (pbk.) –
ISBN 978-0-7748-2871-0 (pdf). – ISBN 978-0-7748-2872-7 (epub)

1. Sex – Religious aspects. I. Young, Pamela Dickey, 1955-, author, editor
II. Trothen, Tracy J. (Tracy Joan), 1963-, author, editor III. Shipley, Heather, 1979-, author, editor IV. Series: Sexuality studies series

| BL65.S4R44 2015 | 201'.7 | C2014-906107-2 |
| | | C2014-906108-0 |

Canadä

UBC Press gratefully acknowledges the financial support for our publishing program of the Government of Canada (through the Canada Book Fund), the Canada Council for the Arts, and the British Columbia Arts Council.

This book has been published with the help of a grant from the Canadian Federation for the Humanities and Social Sciences, through the Awards to Scholarly Publications Program, using funds provided by the Social Sciences and Humanities Research Council of Canada.

UBC Press
The University of British Columbia
2029 West Mall
Vancouver, BC V6T 1Z2
www.ubcpress.ca

Contents

Introduction / 3
Heather Shipley

Part 1: Religion and the Construction of Sexual Minority Rights / 17

1 Beyond Tolerance: Sexual Diversity and Economic Justice / 21
Janet R. Jakobsen

2 "Severely Normal": Sexuality and Religion in Alberta's Bill 44 / 45
Pamela Dickey Young

3 "I'm Not Homophobic, I'm Chinese": Hong Kong Canadian Christians and the Campaign against Same-Sex Marriage / 67
Lee Wing Hin

Part 2: Sexuality and the Construction of Religious Identities / 93

4 Challenging Identity Constructs: The Debate over the Sex Education Curriculum in Ontario / 97
Heather Shipley

5 When Religion Meets Sexuality: Two Tales of Intersection / 119
Andrew Kam-Tuck Yip

6 Women, Sex, and the Catholic Church: The Implications of Domestic Violence for Reproductive Choice / 141
Catherine Holtmann

Part 3: Sexual Bodies/Religious Bodies / 165

7 The Construction of a Sexual Pedagogy: Childhood and Saints in Roman Catholic Discourse / 169
Donald L. Boisvert

8 Corporeal Diversity in the Religion of Sport: The Debate over Enhanced Bodies / 190
Tracy J. Trothen

9 Strong Spirits, Abused Bodies: Social, Political, and Theological Reflections / 220
Nancy Nason-Clark

Conclusion / 241
Pamela Dickey Young

List of Contributors / 247

Index / 250

RELIGION AND SEXUALITY

Introduction

Heather Shipley

Religion and sexuality often appear in conflicting relationships in the public sphere. In the 1990s religious groups were among those who successfully opposed the inclusion of gay men and lesbians in New York City's "Rainbow Curriculum" (Myers 1992). In 2011 the inclusion of gay-straight alliances in the public education system in Ontario under the Accepting Schools Act (Bill 13) (Government of Ontario 2012) sparked a public debate about religion, religious identity, sexual identity, and youthful sexuality. In 2013 the inclusion of sexual minorities in Minnesota's Safe and Supportive Schools Act was the subject of targeted opposition by religious groups that declared the act unconstitutional and by legislators who threatened a ten-hour filibuster that assured the bill would not be voted on or passed in session (Adkins 2013).

Religious voices have also been at the forefront of opposition to same-sex marriage (Dickey Young 2010). In the Canadian context, this opposition was evident in the debate over revision of the Civil Marriage Act in 2005 to include same-sex couples, after cumulative efforts to redefine marriage at the provincial level. It has also been evident in the State of California, which since 2008 has legalized same-sex marriage, overturned the legalization of same-sex marriage, and subsequently seen the ban against same-sex couples declared unconstitutional by a federal judge. Currently, thirty-two American states as well as the District of Columbia have legalized same-sex marriage, and although some states have not legalized it, they recognize same-sex marriages performed in other states.

In 2013 England and Wales passed same-sex marriage legislation, and in 2014 Scotland did likewise. These changes, too, came amid opposition that included religious opposition.

All of these decisions and changes to law and policy have been fraught with controversy and continue to raise debate and discord among groups on all sides of the arguments. As these debates reach the public arena, often the strongest voices heard in opposition to equality rights for sexual minority communities and same-sex couples are religious voices. However, this emphasis on the conflict at the intersection of religion and sexuality can obscure the real issues. In the case of New York City's "Rainbow Curriculum," its creation to foster racial and ethnic respect was overlooked amid charges that a few passages on gay and lesbian identities rendered the curriculum dangerous homosexual propaganda (Myers 1992; Miller 1993). In the case of Ontario's Bill 13, its creation to protect a range of identity categories from discriminatory behaviours in schools, notably from bullying and cyberbullying, was ignored by media coverage that narrowed both the bill and the debate to issues of religion and sexuality and their "inherent" opposition to one another (Artuso 2011; Talaga 2011). In the case of Minnesota's Safe and Supportive Schools Act, its creation to further an anti-bullying agenda was overlooked amid religious opposition to its inclusion of sexual minorities, even though the Safe Schools for All Coalition in Minnesota included religious individuals and groups who supported the act's inclusivity and protection of all students.

Further, the emphasis on religious opposition to sexuality often misrepresents religion. As the Minnesota case makes clear, not all religious individuals or groups are unified in their approach to equality rights based on gender, sexuality, or sexual orientation. Yet moderate or liberal religious voices in support of these modifications are not prominent in public discourse and media (Jordan 2009; Shipley, Chapter 4, this volume). As a consequence, the public debate, and subsequently what looks like a public "contest," over religion and sexuality is narrowly portrayed and essentialized in ways that continue to perpetrate mistaken assumptions about both religion and sexuality, which also furthers the notion that they exist only in tension. However, the voices of those who are both religious and sexually "other" or religious and in support of sexual diversity are becoming louder, even though the assumption is often made that to be religious is to stand in opposition to same-sex relations and sexual diversity.

Religion and sexuality evoke strong responses from individuals and groups because religion and sexuality are usually understood as core components of identity, categories through which individuals identify themselves. Thus debates where religion and sexuality are involved elicit emotional engagement from members of the public and from policy makers and generate wide interest in legal decisions. As the examples above indicate, these controversies are played out in multiple sites of contention, including legal involvement in specific controversies (same-sex marriage); public policy revisions in response to more contemporary frameworks of religious and/or sexual identity (sex education curricula and inclusivity policies); and increasing portrayals of a broad array of subjects pertaining to sexuality and religion through media, film, and popular culture. Public dialogue about such issues demonstrates both the importance of this volume and, more broadly, the ways that Canada and other countries are navigating challenges regarding both religious and sexual diversity in the public eye.

Religious groups have witnessed internal controversy and change regarding sexual diversity and religious ideologies in relation to such topics as same-sex marriage, the sexual accountability of clergy, birth control, abortion, and violence against women and sexual minorities (e.g., Nedelsky and Hutchinson 2008; Holtmann, Chapter 6, this volume; Nason-Clark, Chapter 9, this volume). In some cases, the discussions have divided religious groups dramatically enough to cause schisms, as in the case of the Anglican Church in Canada on the question of the ordination of homosexual clergy. Roman Catholic women who practise birth control are required to construct their religious identities in relation to a church that opposes their contraceptive choices (Dickey Young 2012). Education policies that still seem to discriminate on the basis of sexual orientation have been called into question and, in many cases, revamped as a response to claims of bullying and multiple suicides among sexual minority youth (Friedman 2010).[1]

The academic study of the relationship between religion and sexuality is a relatively new discipline. The regulation of sexuality within the public arena has been strongly influenced – indeed, sometimes controlled – by religious groups and ideologies. In more recent years, and in recent scholarship, a more nuanced analysis of the relationship of religion and sexuality to each other has teased out the ways that various forms of religion and various "non-normative" sexualities do, in fact, coexist, both in an individual's understanding of personal identity and in socially progressive movements that do not take religion and sexuality to be necessarily opposed (Yip et al. 2011; Taylor and Snowdon 2014; Yip, Chapter 5, this volume). The chapters in this collection respond directly and indirectly to policy and media controversies over both religion and sexuality. The authors see the narrow construction of religious identity in media debates about same-sex marriage, sexual minority rights, and sexual identification as highly problematic and inaccurate. They argue that the various forms that religious and sexually diverse engagements take within both public and private spheres offer space for reflecting on the complex articulations of identity as lived and experienced in everyday life.

The diverse scholarship in this collection provides reflection on timely subjects from multiple perspectives based on multiple theoretical approaches. No single, distinctive theoretical approach guides each chapter; rather, the treatment of the topics is inter- and multidisciplinary. There are thematic unities in the collection, including the relationship between religion and the construction of sexual minority rights, the influence of sexuality on the construction of religious identities, and the intertwining of religious and sexual views of the body. These thematic unities are manifested in subthemes such as the complexity of identity negotiation, the diversity of living religion and living sexuality, the limits of multiculturalism, and the question of agency. These subthemes are highlighted as each chapter responds to the intersection of religion and sexuality in public policy and the public imagination. Sometimes these responses expose the problem of the continually recurring negative portrayal of religion in relation to sexual diversity; sometimes they highlight specific forms of religion that still regard sexual diversity as highly problematic.

The terms "sexual diversity" and "religious diversity" can be used in a variety of ways. In the view of this volume's authors, religious diversity is not just about bringing a large number of "different" religions together and comparing them but also about recognizing that within religious traditions much diversity is present. In the countries where the research in this book was conducted – Canada, the United States, and the United Kingdom – there are still large Christian majorities that often become the focus of research, not least because these majorities have made most of the public contributions to discussions of religion and sexuality. Further, most religious traditions are not currently struggling with questions of transsexuality and other more fluid constructions of sexuality.[2] Rather, they are still struggling with traditional sex/gender roles and with same-sex attraction and relationships. Contributors to this volume use and reflect on the categories of religion and sexuality in multifaceted and nuanced ways, challenging the notion that either can be "defined." Instead, their research is informed by the literature on lived religion (e.g., Orsi 2005; McGuire 2008) and on lived sexuality (e.g., Foucault 1978; Weeks 2011). Each case study is intended to compel the reader to reflect on the reasons why these terms cannot – and perhaps should not – be restricted by definitions.

Religious diversity and religious pluralism are frequently debated topics in Canada and elsewhere. Policies regarding the accommodation of religious practices and positive approaches to globalization and multiculturalism have sparked new debates about religion and religious diversity and have often pushed the religious "other" to the forefront of debates about identity, nationhood, and the notion of tolerance of difference (Beaman 2013). Increasingly, scholarship about religion and religious identity has demonstrated that individuals experience their religious ideologies in multiple ways in given timeframes, in given locations, and across their lifespan (e.g., Beckford 2003; Beyer 2006; McGuire 2008). This volume also helps to unravel the complexity of studying diverse identities, as the questions about sexuality and religion presented here are also questions about pluralism, multiculturalism, and diversity.

Discussions and debates about religion and sexuality as sites of contention are found not only in media and public discourses but also in law and policy. Further, university departments of gender and sexuality studies are broadening their scope of studies to address the importance of factors such as regulation, morality, and social construction in the study of gender and sexuality. Clearly, the discussions offered in this volume are timely. Authors explore times, places, and cases where sexuality is a focus of religious discourse and concern, where the formulation of religious and sexual identities impinge on one another, or where public policies intertwine with both sexuality and religion.

The contributors to this volume were invited as a cross-section of a small but growing group of scholars whose work spans the intersection of religion and sexuality. Based on the goal of setting up a genuine dialogue among scholars invited to engage with the topics in a productive way, this volume produces new questions and new approaches concerning both sexual diversity and religious diversity. This volume does not aim to be a complete or final study of all points of intersection between religion and sexuality but rather to analyze a number of specific instances of intersection. It therefore offers a sampling of current debates, reflecting upon the complex ways that religion – particularly as represented in this volume by Christian and Muslim diversity – and sexuality come into one another's orbits.

Authors in this volume build on their previous work to open up new areas for exploration, such as how sexuality is a key component in developing relations of economic justice; the religious, political, and social consequences of our psychic ambivalence about sex; how sexual minority Muslims and Christians are integrating their faith and their sexuality; and the relationship between religious "fanaticism" and the human rights of sexual minorities.

Scholarly studies either blame religion and religious ideologies for the restrictions and norms imposed on gender and sexuality (Short and MacDougall 2010) or leave religion undiscussed when questions of gender and sexuality are at the fore.[3] Chapters in this book illuminate how sexuality challenges religion and how diverse representations and expressions of sexuality can in fact change religion and religious ideology. The fluidity of religious identity and sexual identity in their relationship with one another means that there are no singular mechanisms or models that can be used to define the relationship between the two; rather, ongoing analysis of nuances provides a case-by-case examination of how religion and sexuality shape each other.

The volume has been organized around thematic topics that frame the issues addressed by the authors: religion and the construction of sexual minority rights; sexuality and the construction of religious identities; and sexual bodies/religious bodies. The chapters work together to create a picture of where some of the challenges are being faced in the intersection of religion and sexuality, to challenge commonly held assumptions about the relationships between these two categories of analysis, and to explore lived sexual and religious experiences through understandings of embodiment, thus helping to unravel the relationship between religious identity and sexual identity.

Religion and the Construction of Sexual Minority Rights

The development of sexual minority rights has been a contentious public issue over the past two decades. The first section of this volume provides a comparative jumping-off point to illuminate both the power dynamics inherent in a discussion about sexual minority rights and the relationship of religion to sexual minority rights. Same-sex marriage offers a compelling example of what is at stake for sexual minorities when intimate life is the subject of public debate and controversy. The right of same-sex couples to be legally married is entangled with other debates regarding activism, conservativism, hierarchies among sexual minorities, and what limitations are imposed when same-sex marriage is realized. For some sexual minority activists, rights related to sexual identity should be granted not because one becomes married; rather, these rights should be accessible to individuals regardless of marital status or desire for marriage (see Duggan 2008; Pellegrini 2009). In cases where the legalization of same-sex marriage or the redefinition of marriage to include same-sex couples has provided a public arena for debates about family, "morality," and the "clash" of religion and sexual diversity, the ways that such changes create a new, disadvantaged group of sexual minorities have not been prevalent in public discourse.

In Chapter 1, Janet Jakobsen challenges readers by asking what we are moving toward if we are moving beyond tolerance? Jakobsen suggests that it is time to move from an ideal of religious or sexual tolerance to an ideal of religious or sexual freedom when discussing rights claims and international politics. Jakobsen argues that it is time to think critically about how economic justice (or a lack thereof) is implicated in debates about religious and sexual diversity. Assessing current policies in the US context, Jakobsen critiques the continued reliance on stereotypical gender roles, which correspondingly reinstate economic disparities that mark initiatives such as the Office of Faith-Based and Neighborhood Partnerships (White House 2009).

In Chapter 2, Pamela Dickey Young argues that Alberta's Bill 44, which in 2009 modified the Alberta Human Rights Act, helps to reinforce heteronormativity by reading sexuality and sexual orientation as problematic. By inserting education policy into a human rights context, Bill 44 creates a human rights breach in instances when a teacher includes religion, sexuality, or sexual orientation in the classroom without providing parents with advance notice. Dickey Young contends that this bill was meant to solve a political problem, not an educational or human rights problem, and was intended as an "olive branch" to religious people and conservative voters.

In Chapter 3, Lee Wing Hin traces the deployment of the languages of multiculturalism, race, ethnicity, and colonialism in the same-sex marriage debate by Hong Kong Christians in Canada, arguing that some constituencies claiming to speak for all Hong Kong Canadians used normative discourse to argue for their right to be heard in order to promote what they believed was the one religiously and sexually moral truth. Troubling, from Lee's perspective, was an accompanying narrative that positioned Chinese immigration to Canada as part of a divine plan and that denied the brutal realities of Canadian immigration policy of the nineteenth century.

The authors in this section negotiate multiple possible dialogues about the ways that religion and sexual diversity interact. Policy decisions do not exist in a vacuum, devoid of human interaction, but are developed within particular social and political contexts. Further, a community's narrative about its own identity within a nation might not consider the actuality of policies that its members are required to negotiate as citizens. And although this volume focuses on religion and sexuality, the reality is that these two categories are never the "only" subjects implicated at any given time; the rights of sexual minorities to recognition, inclusivity, and access are always also about the rights to citizenship and economic and distributive justice.

Sexuality and the Construction of Religious Identities

Questioning the relationship between religion and sexuality in policy, law, and politics requires fleshing out the categories and the complexity of identity construction. For example, research on religion, gender, and sexuality among youth in Canada demonstrates the tension between rigid dictates about religious identity and the lived experience of religious identity for youth (Dickey Young and Shipley 2014). For many, the expression of their lived religious identity is often not institutionally approved, yet it is this day-to-day experience of "being religious" that informs religious individuality in relation to other categories of identity, such as gender and sexuality (ibid.). It is by challenging assumptions about identity categories and rigidity that a robust understanding of the complexity of both religious identity and sexual identity becomes possible. The contributors to this section challenge assumptions made in policy or discourse about the construction of identities and dig into lived experiences of religious and sexual identities.

In Chapter 4, Heather Shipley focuses on the changes to the Ontario sex education curriculum proposed in 2010, the ensuing controversy in the media, and the subsequent hold that was placed on the proposed changes pending further review. Because there were religious groups in opposition to the proposed changes to sex education, the debate essentialized religion as being opposed to queer sexual identities, thus creating a false dichotomy that disregarded the diversity of options both for religious identities and choices and for sexual identities and choices.

In Chapter 5, Andrew Kam-Tuck Yip draws on primary research in the United Kingdom, emphasizing that identity politics is more than a human political strategy for resistance and change. In the context of the diktat of sex only within marriage, Yip challenges the apparent dichotomy between religious repression and secular freedom and suggests that identity politics has salient spiritual significance and symbolism because sexual minority religious actors draw on the power of their religious understandings for encouragement of individual and collective agency for change.

In Chapter 6, Catherine Holtmann emphasizes the importance of exploring women's lived religious experiences and describes strategies used by the women in her research when they faced issues of sexuality and social justice. These women questioned official religious views of sexuality and privileged their own and others' lived experiences in understanding sexuality. Holtmann fleshes out the experiential reality for women of faith in her study, who negotiated their perceptions of religiosity and sexuality based on personal experience and understanding, not on dogma or doctrine.

Although religious and sexual identities are constructed as being in opposition to one another, and are then regulated as though they were inherently oppositional, the exploration of identity continues to demonstrate that individual experiences of religion and religiosity are fluid, not dichotomously fixed. Further, as illustrated by Yip, the assumption that secularity is a space of freedom has also been proven untrue. The push for social justice is not contained solely within the "neutral" secular sphere, and the secular sphere is not in fact necessarily an inclusive or accepting space (Taylor and Peter 2011).

Sexual Bodies/Religious Bodies

Embodiment is an important and necessary topic when one examines the variety of ways that complex identity markers such as religion and sexuality are lived and experienced. The proposed Charter of Values (Bill 60) in Quebec is evidence of how the regulation of religion and religiosity implicates bodies, particularly where religious "freedom" is directly linked to the regulation of women's bodies and women's clothing. Bill 60, in its proposed exalting of the "secular" public sphere, restricts religious identity expressions, predominantly for Muslim women. Exploring how bodies are the subject of "oppression" versus "freedom" regarding religion and sexuality, authors in this section question the ways that bodies are subjected to regulation and to assumptions about religion and embodiment.

In Chapter 7, Donald Boisvert explores the way that liminal teenage bodies are constructed as dangerous and oversexualized yet also chaste. Boisvert argues that in North American Catholic culture, these bodies are moulded and tamed through devotion to adolescent saints. Boisvert's chapter explores the conflict between Catholic teaching regarding sexualized bodies and the experience of teenage sexual identity in relation to Catholic saints.

In Chapter 8, Tracy Trothen shows how the intersection between techno-science, sport, and religion has ambivalent implications for the understanding of embodiment and sexuality. Examining the normative assumptions about sexuality and gender that are operative in elite sport, Trothen reflects on the ways that female and gay athletes disrupt both masculine and heteronormative assumptions about what being an athlete "looks like." Drawing a link between sport and religion, Trothen argues that embodiment diversity within sport offers transformative possibilities.

In Chapter 9, Nancy Nason-Clark focuses on domestic violence within faith communities, outlining how her research on domestic violence against women in religious homes, including sexual violence, makes the very real physical body of a battered woman a site for religious dispute. Nason-Clark offers a nuanced perspective on the social, political, and theological underpinnings and assertions that impact and define abuse within communities of faith.

Authors in this final section demonstrate both the complexity of the relationship between religion and sexual bodies and how this embodiment is necessarily embedded with the assumption that religion is oppressive and that secularism is inclusive. By teasing out the ways that normative bodily assumptions are regularly disrupted by lived religious, gendered, and sexual realities, this section offers a window into the multiple possibilities of religious and sexual embodiment. Correspondingly, policies of bodily regulation often have a gendered impact, with women's bodies as the frequent sites of regulation, within both secular and religious bodily policies.

These three thematic frameworks denote key questions about the relationship between sexual diversity and religious diversity, drawing on important, timely, and contentious issues to elaborate the complexity of the study of religion and sexuality. The diversity of the methodological and theoretical approaches of the contributors allows for a nuanced analysis and for the development of new ways of thinking through the topics of study in this volume. Multifaceted views of the ways that religion interacts with sexuality are offered in chapters on topics such as religion and reproductive rights, sexual violence, and the construction of sexual identities. Authors analyze not just religious "positions" but also the lives of religious people who challenge traditional religious views of sexual identity. This work contributes to discussions about religion and sexuality in Canada and abroad by providing several perspectives on the relationships between the various topics in this volume. Comparative analysis with the United States and the United Kingdom provides important reference points by which to locate Canada in the debates about religion and sexuality.

Following on Jakobsen's argument in Chapter 1 that we must consider what we are moving toward, many authors in this volume employ queer theory to challenge assumptions and stereotypes evident in the case studies presented here. The queering of the topics that they discuss provides conceptually diverse spaces from which to view possibilities regarding the study of religion and sexuality. This volume seeks to open up new avenues of interrogation in the study of religion and sexuality and to expose their complexity.

Notes

The editors wish to thank the Social Sciences and Humanities Research Council of Canada (SSHRC) for funding the workshop that gave rise to this book. Some of the contributors also received funding from the Religion and Diversity Project (http://religionanddiversity.ca), a SSHRC-funded research initiative housed at the University of Ottawa, Ontario. We also wish to thank two anonymous reviewers of the manuscript for UBC Press, who offered important suggestions and critiques that helped to strengthen the volume as a whole.

1 This connection between bullying and suicide was represented by the death of Tyler Clementi, a Rutgers University student who committed suicide after his roommate streamed footage of him engaged in homosexual relations on YouTube (Friedman 2010).
2 See, for example, the same-sex marriage debate in Canada (Dickey Young 2012), where none of the religious groups involved discussed transsexuality.
3 Although some research about gender and sexuality also explicitly reflects on religion – whether positively, neutrally, or negatively – much research about gender and sexuality builds more specifically on psychology, sociology, feminist theories, and so on. The subfield that combines religion with gender/sexuality is a much smaller discipline.

References

Adkins, J. 2013. Catholic Church Favors Anti-bullying Efforts – Just Not So-Called "Safe and Supportive Schools Act." *Minnesota Post*, 24 April. http://www.minnpost.com/community-voices/2013/04/catholic-church-favors-anti-bullying-efforts-just-not-so-called-safe-and-su.

Artuso, A. 2011. Religious Group Attacks Anti-bullying Law – Says McGuinty Not a Good Catholic. *Sault Ste. Marie Star*, 7 December. http://www.saultstar.com/2011/12/07/religious-group-attacks-anti-bullying-law-says-mcguinty-not-a-good-catholic.

Beaman, L. 2013. The Will to Religion: Obligatory Religious Citizenship. *Critical Research on Religion* 1 (2): 141-57.

Beckford, J. 2003. *Social Theory and Religion*. Cambridge: Cambridge University Press.

Beyer, P. 2006. *Religions in Global Society*. London: Routledge.

Dickey Young, P. 2010. Taking Account of Religion in Canada: The Debates over Gay and Lesbian Marriage. *Studies in Religion/Sciences Religieuses* 39 (3): 333-61.

–. 2012. *Religion, Sex, and Politics: Christian Churches and Same-Sex Marriage in Canada*. Winnipeg: Fernwood.

Dickey Young, P., and H. Shipley. 2014, in press. Belief, Not Religion: Youth Negotiations of Religious Identity in Canada. In *Handbook of Child and Youth Studies*, ed. J. Wyn and H. Cahill. New York: Springer.

Duggan, L. 2008. Beyond Same-Sex Marriage. *Studies in Gender and Sexuality* 9 (2): 155-57.

Foucault, M. 1978. *The History of Sexuality.* Vol. 1, *An Introduction.* Trans. R. Hurley. New York: Random House.

Friedman, E. 2010. Victim of Secret Dorm Sex Tape Posts Facebook Goodbye, Jumps to His Death. *ABC News,* 29 September. http://abcnews.go.com/US/victim-secret-dorm-sex-tape-commits-suicide/story?id=11758716.

Government of Ontario. 2012. *Bill 13: Accepting Schools Act.* http://ontla.on.ca/web/bills/bills_detail.do?locale=en&BillID=2549.

Jordan, M. 2009. Respondent: Marriage, Civil Unions, Domestic Partnerships, and Political Progress and/or Setbacks. Paper presented at the Annual Conference of the American Academy of Religion, Montreal, Quebec, November.

McGuire, M.B. 2008. *Lived Religion: Faith and Practice in Everyday Life.* New York: Oxford University Press.

Miller, J.J. 1993. The Rest of the "Rainbow" Curriculum. *Wall Street Journal,* 10 February. http://www.heymiller.com/2010/08/rainbow-curriculum.

Myers, S.L. 1992. How a "Rainbow Curriculum" Turned into Fighting Words. *New York Times,* 13 December. http://www.nytimes.com/1992/12/13/weekinreview/ideas-trends-how-a-rainbow-curriculum-turned-into-fighting-words.html.

Nedelsky, J., and R. Hutchinson. 2008. Clashes of Principle and the Possibility of Dialogue: A Case Study of Same-Sex Marriage in the United Church of Canada. In *Law and Religious Pluralism in Canada,* ed. R. Moon, 41-64. Vancouver: UBC Press.

Orsi, R. 2005. *Between Heaven and Earth: The Religious Worlds People Make and the Scholars Who Study Them.* Princeton, NJ: Princeton University Press.

Pellegrini, A. 2009. Sexual Freedom, Religious Exemptions, and Secular Citizenship: Constitutional and Civic Challenges in the Contemporary United States. Paper presented in the lecture series Critical Thinkers in Religion, Law and Social Theory, University of Ottawa, 23 October.

Short, D., and B. MacDougall. 2010. Religion-Based Claims for Impinging on Queer Citizenship. *Dalhousie Law Journal* 33 (3): 133-60.

Talaga, T. 2011. Anti-bullying Bill a Front for "Sex Ed" Agenda, Groups Say. *Toronto Star,* 6 December. http://www.thestar.com/news/canada/politics/article/1097682-anti-bullying-bill-a-front-for-sex-ed-agenda-groups-say.

Taylor, C., and T. Peter. 2011. "We are not aliens, we're people, and we have rights": Canadian Human Rights Discourse and High School Climate for LGBTQ Students. *Canadian Review of Sociology* 48 (3): 275-313.

Taylor, Y., and R. Snowdon. 2014. Mapping Queer, Mapping Me: Visualising Queer Religious Identity. In *Globalized Religion and Sexual Identity: Contexts, Contestations, Voices,* ed. H. Shipley, 295-312. Leiden: Brill.

Weeks, J. 2011. *The Languages of Sexuality.* New York: Routledge.

White House. 2009. "Obama Announces White House Office of Faith-Based and Neighborhood Partnerships." Press release. 5 February. http://www.whitehouse.gov/the_press_office/ObamaAnnouncesWhiteHouseOfficeofFaith-basedandNeighborhoodPartnerships.

Yip, A., S. Page, and M. Keenan. 2011. *Religion, Youth and Sexuality: Selected Key Findings from a Multi-faith Exploration*. Nottingham, UK: University of Nottingham.

PART 1
Religion and the Construction of Sexual Minority Rights

THE ISSUE OF RIGHTS is very complex. All the authors in this section, in various ways, are clear that rights-based arguments are inadequate and dangerous if they do not take into account wider contextual factors, including both the function and distribution of power, which are connected with systemic valuing or devaluing, and the interdependence of life. For example, as Janet Jakobsen points out in Chapter 1, autonomy cannot be adequately understood in only an individualistic sense; one's rights do not exist without reference to those of others. The question of whose interests are served by any particular normative definition or prioritizing of rights (either implicit or explicit) is one that can be read in the background of each of these important essays.

The tendency of rights discourses to be used to serve operative interests is well demonstrated in this section. Jakobsen examines the use of the rhetoric of equality and openness by the United States government, concluding that regardless of this rhetoric approaches to gender and sexuality are informed by a normative conservative Christian framework. In Chapter 2, Pamela Dickey Young critiques the Albertan political claim that Bill 44 is merely an attempt to respond both to the rights of those discriminated against on the basis of sexual orientation and to the rights of conservative religious parents regarding their child's sex and religious education. In Chapter 3, Lee Wing Hin argues that in the 2003-05 campaigns against same-sex marriage, constituencies claiming to speak for all Hong Kong Canadians used multicultural normative discourse to argue for their right to be heard in order to promote what they believed was the one religious and sexually moral truth. Each of these chapters illuminates the importance of rights particularly for the marginalized and also the inadequacy of rights-based arguments when they are built on assumptive values that privilege one group at the expense of another.

This epistemological privileging is typically built on presumptions of one truth, fostering us-them binaries that discourage and punish diversity outside of the norm. The insight of feminist, postmodern, and queer theories that truth is dynamic, partial, and perspectival is threaded throughout these chapters. Additional themes related to rights discourses include the systemic power issues of racism and sexism, constructions of multiculturalism, neoliberalism, normative definitions of Christian-cum-secular family values, and the camouflaging of religious diversity. Also connected to these themes are the very significant questions of identity and moral agency that are raised again and again throughout this anthology.

Here, I offer a brief word about the usefulness of this section in teaching: when put in dialogue with each other, this collection of essays can generate vigorous classroom conversation not only about the more visible themes but also about other inferred threads. In addition, hints of controversy in these chapters provide fertile ground for classroom debate; for example, just how pervasive is Canada's new homonormativity, discussed by Dickey Young and by Lee? And, connected to this theme, what are the limitations of Canadian multiculturalism?

Jakobsen examines the links between sexual diversity and economic justice. Building on her previously developed argument that we must move from religious tolerance to religious freedom, Jakobsen asks why public discourse in the United States both devalues and overvalues sex and sexuality – why sex has become the location of moral preoccupation.

Refuting the common assertion that "religious regulation" by a normative conservative Christianity is the single main cause of the United States' national sexual preoccupation, Jakobsen argues that the problem is rooted as much in "secular freedom," albeit a secularism that depends on Christianity for its identity. Drawing on Foucauldian insights about discourses of political biopower and economic free markets, she explores the complexity of moral agency in the context of highly regulated individual sexual freedom in the United States.

Freedom, Jakobsen argues, is constructed in a manner that reinforces the status quo's hierarchies, which maintain complementary gender relationships and the marginalization of sexual and racial minorities, among others. Jakobsen concludes that freedom is insufficient as a moral criterion; an expansive view of justice is necessary to address the causal dynamics undergirding oppression, including the maintenance of us-them dynamics that subvert sexual minority rights.

Religious studies scholar Pamela Dickey Young examines Alberta's Bill 44 and reactions to it. Passed in June 2009, Bill 44 was to codify, finally, that sexual orientation was a prohibited basis for discrimination. But the bill also curiously – or not so curiously, as Dickey Young's analysis makes clear – includes provisions regarding parental rights and education on sexuality and religion. Dickey Young identifies several issues generated by the bill and the highly charged reactions to it. These issues are related to power and normative constructions of both religion and sexuality. Her chapter is about who has rights, what rights, and whose rights are most or least valid in the contemporary context. Dickey Young uncovers normative values by asking who is privileged enough to define the issues and decide what diversity is permitted. As part of this analysis, she includes a discussion of religious diversity and whose religion or version of religion counts as normal, true, or valid. Dickey Young ends with a proposal for a vision of "deep equality" that embraces sexual and religious diversity.

Lee considers an example of the commitment of a group's members to regulating sex in order to preserve and further what "they" perceive as the one true value system and moral code. Lee examines the protests of Hong Kong Canadians against the 2005 Canadian legalization of same-sex marriage. While pointing to the complicated and important issues of racism and colonialism as they relate to sexual and religious diversity, Lee raises the question of how ethnically defined communities can gain voice and power without subsuming their own diversity and without claiming particular values as normative for their community.

Unmasking claims of one homogeneous Hong Kong Canadian voice and identity, Lee finds that the organized protest campaigns were motivated by a missionary drive to save the nation through a conservative, evangelical, Protestant re-Christianization. Protest leaders claimed that Chinese people universally condemned homosexuality and same-sex unions, which they regarding as counter to salvation. Such claims of homogeneity and deliberate attempts to gain power through appeals to Canadian multicultural policy were seen as justified by "their" faith. Lee uncovers causal dynamics through an exploration of the historically informed identities of Hong Kong Canadians, tracing the historic Canadian colonial exploitation of Chinese labour and relating this to the ongoing effects of religion as a tool of colonization.

Lee's chapter introduces the reader to a multilayered example of the tendency to locate sin and salvation in regulated and exclusionary sex norms, as well as the tendency to repeat exploitative power dynamics that are justified by claims of access to "the" truth.

– Tracy J. Trothen

1

Beyond Tolerance
SEXUAL DIVERSITY AND ECONOMIC JUSTICE

Janet R. Jakobsen

When it comes to public life and social policy, Canada can seem to be ahead of the United States on a number of fronts: healthcare, gun control, and well-being more generally. Perhaps most of all, when viewed from the United States, it looks like Canada is significantly advanced on issues of tolerance, pluralism, and diversity. As a scholar, I know that this is undoubtedly a romanticized view (and I do ask that all Canadians go easy on those of us from the United States for whom Canada provides an enabling fantasy – don't burst our bubble too quickly). Yet tolerance has it limits, and in the workshop on which this volume is based, authors were asked to move "beyond" tolerance, accommodation, and pluralism, a move with which I wholeheartedly concur. So if we move "beyond" the limits of contemporary discourses about both religious and sexual diversity, what do we move toward?

In our co-authored book *Love the Sin: Sexual Regulation and the Limits of Religious Tolerance* (2003), Ann Pellegrini and I suggest that we might move from religious tolerance to religious freedom. In this chapter, I further explore the question of freedom – its possibilities and limits – in the hope of moving toward something that, in conjunction with a reimagined, queer freedom, we might call justice. Throughout this chapter, I draw on the resources of queer theory to explore the meaning of basic values, like freedom and justice, in the hope that queer versions of these concepts might provide some newly inspiring vision.

The questions so helpfully posed at the workshop were: What do we learn by tarrying at the intersection of religious and sexual diversity? Why hold a conference that ties together questions about religious diversity with those about sexual politics?

There is good reason to think that gender and sexuality do play a major role in debates about religious diversity and in shaping religious communities. Gender and sexuality tend to appear in such debates as crucial mediating points at the boundaries of religious difference. Examples abound of the invocation of gender and sexuality as proof of religious difference – whether at the abstract level of the discussion of religious pluralism, like Huntington's (2005) concern about the reproductive practices of Catholic immigrants in his defence of a Protestant culture in the United States, or at the local level of boundary negotiations over public space and Hasidic Jewish practice in Brooklyn, New York, or at the governmental level of the possibility of sharia courts in Canada to adjudicate family law (Pierre-Pierre 1997). Whatever the context, gender and sexuality are likely to be a part of discussions of religious difference (Emon 2010). But as Heather Shipley shows in Chapter 4 of this volume, gender and sexuality can also provide sites for presuming religious convergence across difference, where an assumed consonance between religiosity and sexual conservatism unites different religions while dividing the religious (and supposedly sexually conservative) from the secular (and supposedly sexually liberal). Whether in its differentiating or uniting aspect, sexuality is presumed to have a special role in revealing "the truth" of religious difference – much as Foucault (1980) noted that sexuality provides the truth of the self in modernity.

In US politics, the importance of the intersection of religion and sexuality has long been evident. Since the late 1970s this intersection has been understood to be inhabited by religious conservatives and conservative politicians; but if one considers these social relations more carefully, it is possible to see that the politics of religion and sexuality are important to actors across the political spectrum. For example, the administration of President Barack Obama staked a claim to this intersection from its earliest days in 2009. Specifically, the ties between religious diversity and sexual politics were no further away than in his administration's initial charge to its Office of Faith-Based and Neighborhood Partnerships. This office was a continuation and even expansion of the program that the administration of President George W. Bush had established as the Office of Faith-Based and Community Initiatives (itself an expansion of the "charitable choice" in the 1996 "welfare reform" bill, signed by President Bill Clinton). The press release announcing the charge to the office in January 2009 tied questions of religion, gender, and sexuality to economic well-being, as well as national security.

The overall charge to the Office of Faith-Based and Neighborhood Partnerships was the task of supporting both secular and religious community groups in their "work on behalf of Americans committed to improving their communities no matter their religious or political beliefs" (White House 2009). The office was also conceptualized as having an advisory role on policy. Moreover, as the charge to this office articulated, this expansion into the administration's development of policy had a broad reach, including both domestic and foreign policy issues:

- The Office's top priority will be making community groups an integral part of our economic recovery and poverty a burden fewer have to bear when recovery is complete.
- It will be one voice among several in the administration that will look at how we support women and children, address teenage pregnancy, and reduce the need for abortion.
- The Office will strive to support fathers who stand by their families, which involves working to get young men off the streets and into well-paying jobs, and encouraging responsible fatherhood.
- Finally, beyond American shores this Office will work with the National Security Council to foster interfaith dialogue with leaders and scholars around the world. (Ibid.)

The charge begins with the top governmental priority in early 2009 of addressing economic recovery, and the Obama administration takes the additional step of directly naming poverty as a problem, but this agenda is followed by "key priorities" that are explicitly related to gender and sexuality: addressing "teenage pregnancy," abortion reduction, and support for fathers "who stand by their families." Interestingly, Obama is hoping to bring men more directly into the question of gender and sexuality by adding the explicit interpellation of "fathers" to the feminine – and sometimes troublesomely feminist – politics of abortion. And in the cases of support for "women and children" and of support for (good) "fathers," we see an approach that Obama used at the beginning of his first term: the creation of a new policy by combining aspects of the policies advocated by what are understood to be the two "sides" of American politics. Although Americans cannot, four decades after *Roe v. Wade,* agree on the legality of abortion, Obama posits that they should be able to agree that the world would be better if fewer women needed to have abortions. Importantly, unlike in the case of "responsible fatherhood," where a means of supporting fathers is identified, the explicit means of reducing abortion is not mentioned because there are radical political differences on method. Some advocate abortion reduction through universal sex education and readily available contraception, as well as economic possibilities for women so that their childbearing is not constrained by dire economic circumstances, whereas others advocate traditional family values, promotion of abstinence and marriage, and restrictions on the availability of abortion as ways to reduce the number of abortions performed each year. In the case of responsible fatherhood, the means of supporting fathers is identified as getting them off of the streets and into well-paying jobs, thus bringing together traditional liberal support for jobs programs and more conservative support for the "traditional" two-parent family (ibid.).

Despite the sense that each policy brings together liberal and conservative elements, the overall effect of linking the two policies is to create a traditional vision of American gender roles, family structures, and their implications. Obama's policy exhibits explicit gendering in that it directs different initiatives at women and men, and in its explicitness the policy is also traditional: women are connected to children and need to be supported so that abortions are not necessary, but they apparently don't need well-paying jobs, unlike the fathers. (Queer and transgendered people are nowhere named.) In the space of this initial charge to the Office of Faith-Based and Neighborhood Partnerships, the move is relatively swift from a new recognition of the importance of community-based advocates "no matter their religious or political beliefs" to "traditional" family values, which are often associated with conservative Christianity through organizations like Focus on the Family. These values mandate a two-parent family of distinctly differentiated genders, with the father working and the mother caring for children; although she may work outside the home, there is no mention of government support for this activity.

As the charge continues, we also move very rapidly from economic recovery through family values to the somewhat startling inclusion of the National Security Council despite the focus on "neighborhood" partnerships. How is it that the domestic (in every sense of the word) gender normativity of the office is tied to what the administration here calls "the world beyond our shores"? The Obama administration's approach is undoubtedly different from that of the Bush administration. The turn toward interfaith dialogue instead of a "crusade" for freedom and the directive to take up dialogue with both "leaders" (presumably religious leaders?) and "scholars" (perhaps thought of as secular?) marks the greater openness to the world that many commentators saw in Obama's 2009 speech in Cairo.[1] But the overall framework instituted by the administration maintains the Christian hegemony of the neoliberal world order. In particular, the dialogue model for interrelation across religious difference claims to be based in equality and openness but is actually framed by a Christian understanding.

The model of interfaith dialogue offers negotiation between different "faiths," a view of religion that mirrors the Christian emphasis on belief as definitive of religion. If, however, practice or land is the basis for one's religion, dialogue might not be the way to approach conflict. For interfaith dialogues, the issue is talking through beliefs rather than, for example, negotiating about land rights. As with the secular calendar, which is at once used across cultures and specifically Christian, these assumptions make the claim of the office to be open to participation "no matter" what into a claim that is simultaneously universalist and Christian. In other words, despite its proclaimed openness, the charge places issues of gender and sexuality and of religious diversity into a traditional and normative Christian framework. And, indeed, despite early controversies about the overwhelming Christian nature of the President's Advisory Council on Faith-Based and Neighborhood Partnerships, the membership of the council remains predominantly Christian.[2]

This example shows that when it comes to US public policy, gender and sexuality are deeply tied to religion and to a particular vision of religious diversity. Obama's enactment of a policy that supports normative gender and sexual arrangements in a "faith-based" context while expounding a vision of diversity that nonetheless manages to maintain the central position of Christianity suggests why a volume that explicitly ties the intersection of sexuality and religion to questions of diversity might be illuminating. It also invites us to move "beyond" a type of tolerance and accommodation that promises openness while maintaining the dominant position of specifically Christian traditions.

What's Wrong with Tolerance?

In *Love the Sin,* Ann Pellegrini and I explore the ethos of tolerance that is applied to sexuality and crystallized in the catchphrase "love the sinner, hate the sin," which is widely used, even by US politicians at the highest levels of government (Jakobsen and Pellegrini 2003, 2). We also ask about the relationship of this ethos to the religious freedom that is supposed to be the hallmark of the United States. There is good reason to believe that the treatment of religious practice in US law is more like "tolerance" than like freedom, with Christianity maintaining a central position in relation to which "other" religions are variously marginalized and tolerated.

As the catchphrase "love the sinner, hate the sin" shows, gay, lesbian, queer, and transgendered people are positioned not as subjects of freedom but as the objects of tolerance. They are positioned specifically through the invocation of a regulatory religious ethics that promises the "love" so often offered by the Christian right – and even by those not so far to the right – even as the "sin" is "hated." This hatred of the "sin" moves quite easily and quickly to denial of people's basic rights as either citizens or human beings, if not to outright hatred of people associated with the "sin."

Pellegrini and I argue that this slide is so easy because tolerance doesn't really fight the problem of hatred; it maintains the structures of hierarchy and discrimination on which hatred is based. Tolerance establishes a hierarchical relation between a dominant centre and its margin, between those who tolerate and those who are tolerated: specifically, tolerance is structured to create and reinforce the idea of an "us" that tolerates "them" (all those who can be positioned as "other.")

This us-them dynamic establishes the "general public" of the United States, a group that supposedly includes everyone but that actually includes the perceived majority, positioned at the centre, with the tolerated minorities positioned at the margins. Whenever "we" are asked to tolerate "them," this same margin-centre relationship comes into play. As Pellegrini and I conclude, "Being the object of tolerance does not represent full inclusion in American life, but rather a grudging form of acceptance in which the boundary between 'us' and 'them' remains clear, sometimes dangerously so" (Jakobsen and Pellegrini 2003, 52).

As a result, the religious tolerance offered in the United States shades easily from the disestablishment and free exercise that are provided by the First Amendment to the US Constitution into a hierarchical religious tolerance in which Christian norms and values form the framework for secular democracy in the United States. Berger (2010) provides a similar analysis of the limits of Canadian legal promises of tolerance. He points out that the promise that you can participate as equals as long as you adhere to the specific values of the Canadian legal system is contradictory: immigrants can be equal to Canadians only if they live according to values that are Canadian. But what happens when these values are not the values shared by immigrants? What if, for example, immigrants are perceived to be intolerant? In such cases, the limits of tolerance are reached. As Berger (ibid., 108) argues, "Law tolerates that which is different only as long as it is not so different that it challenges the organizing norms, commitments, practices, and symbols of the Canadian constitutional rule of law."

As Pellegrini and I show through readings of both court cases and cultural controversies, the same dynamic holds true in the United States. Subscribers to non-Christian values are (sometimes) tolerated if these values, whether we are speaking of sexuality or religion, do not challenge the dominant frame of Christian presumption in public life. For example, one can be Jewish and thrive in the United States if, as the US Supreme Court has ruled, this does not mean that one wants to wear a yarmulke with one's Air Force uniform (*Goldman v. Weinberger* 1986) or to open one's shop on the Christian Sabbath in violation of local Sunday closing laws (*Braunfeld v. Brown* 1961) (Jakobsen and Pellegrini 2003, 110). This type of boundary setting, in which some religious practices exceed the boundaries of tolerance, means that members of religious minorities often face a daily dilemma over how much of their religious "difference" they can or should enact in public.

Proclaiming openness while setting precise limits to this openness is the "trick" of liberal tolerance (Kazanjian 2003). For those who don't share "American" values, neither the law nor the supposed openness of tolerance actually protects them *in their difference*. They are subjects of law and tolerance only in so far as they fit within the predominant frame of values. This trick means that some values (i.e., those held by the majority) are more equal than others.

In contrast, we argue that queers are not deviants to be tolerated. Queers, immigrants, and other "minorities" are free and equal subjects, along with those who claim to love them even as they would deny them equal rights. They are subjects not of tolerance but of freedom and justice.

Sex in Public

But what do freedom and justice mean, particularly if these values are to be something other than liberal values that apply to all people *until they don't?*

To answer this question, we need to think more about sex and its intersection with religion. Specifically, why is it that questions of sexual difference and diversity are such flashpoints in many parts of the world today, including both the United States and Canada? If one traces the arc of US political controversies over the past thirty years, it seems as though sex and issues related to sex – gay rights, sexual and reproductive health, gender conformity, and family relations – are the driving force of US politics.

The typical explanation for why sexuality is so central to US politics has to do with the particular religious heritage of the United States and with the ways that religion continues to play an extensive role in American politics, well beyond its role in most other industrialized countries.[3] In this view, religiously motivated repression is the root of the problem, and freedom from religion is the answer to the problem. This traditional view plays into a larger Enlightenment narrative in which freedom from religion brings about human liberation. In contrast to this view, however, I have argued extensively that the problem is as much secular as it is religious (Jakobsen 2005, 2010). Specifically, secular values – like the freedom from religion promised in the Enlightenment and the "justice for all" promised in US culture[4] – are a driving force behind sexual regulation in the United States. Thus, if we hope to shift sexual politics, we need to reimagine these values rather than simply assert them over those expounded by conservative religious advocates. Fortunately, sex – including its relation to religion – can provide a fertile ground for this reimagining.

To better understand the forces driving US sexual politics, it is helpful to begin with the factors other than religion that might contribute to the US obsession with sexuality. Queer studies scholars have tracked this recurrent obsession, showing how sex has repeatedly been deployed to create "moral panics" that regulate not just sexual activity but also relations of race and class in the United States and the boundaries of the nation itself. Sex has worked its magic as a focal point for regulation in issues like public health, welfare reform, immigration, and militarism. Both Duggan (2000) and Ferguson (2003) have shown, for example, how the violence of race relations is maintained – given both emotional charge and legitimacy – through a discourse of sexuality. Whether it is the deeply sexualized violence of lynching or the effects of coldly analytic sociological studies that picture African Americans as sexually deviant and unable to form "normal" families, racism depends on sexuality for proof of deviance. Shah (2005) has shown how the legal apparatus of sodomy prosecutions could be deployed to manage immigrant communities, establishing both racial boundaries and the boundaries of citizenship. And Duggan (2004) has shown how sex is integral to US conflicts that fuel neoliberal economic policies and intensify income inequality.

This combination of gender, race, class, and sex has worked so powerfully that in the 1990s a major economic change like "welfare reform," which marked the full embrace of neoliberalism on the part of the US government, could be carried out through a discourse that rarely mentioned economics. The debate did obsessively discuss "teenage mothers," a euphemism for young, poor women of colour who are sexually active. At one point in the development of the political momentum for "reform," President Bill Clinton claimed that "teenage mothers" were the greatest threat facing the United States as a nation (West 2000, 138). In this case, Clinton gladly deployed the discourse of sexual conservatism, which was later used against him and has continued to be used by conservatives up to the present moment.

The recurrent obsession with sex in public life is one side of an American ambivalence that moves between the obsessive publicity of sex and the utter privatization of sexuality. As Berlant and Duggan (2001, 5) have argued, US public discourse "simultaneously overvalues and devalues sex and sexuality," but the devaluation is as misleading about the role of sex and values in US public life as is the overvaluation. Even when not done in the context of a moral panic, the regulation of sexuality is a central focus of the government and is enacted both through laws that are directly concerned with sexuality, such as marriage laws and laws regulating commercial sex, and through laws that depend on sexual relations more indirectly, such as immigration laws based on "family reunification." In the end, denying the importance of sex in public does not diminish the cultural and political effects of sex, but it does make these effects more opaque and less open to critique.

Sexual politics drives both "culture wars" and political campaigns, but there are other ways of understanding sex, particularly in relation to values. Specifically, sex can be a site of moral concern without being required to carry the burdens of the nation as a whole.

Why Sex? Why Religion?

If religious repression is not the sole cause of moral panics, why is there such a frequent focus on sex in US public life? After all, sex has not always been the central site of moral concern, even in the Christian areas of the world that serve as genealogical sources for public life in the United States.[5] As Foucault (1980) so aptly narrates, a new moral order appears in modernity, one that sets up a particular type of moral problem, that of normativity. When it comes to sex, for example, marriage was long the norm in terms that we would now define statistically, but it was not the ideal of sexual morality in these Christian societies; the ideal was celibacy in monastic life. The modern convergence between norm and ideal sets up a particular type of moral problem, one where normative discipline becomes the centrepiece of moral life.

This new moral order is tied to new, specifically modern, forms of governance through what Foucault (1980, 140; 1991, 98ff) terms "biopower." No longer is the Crown's capacity to threaten subjects with death the centre of the state's power; rather, in the modern period, it is control over life, over the means by which life is produced, that maintains the state. Managing the population's activities is what is required, and normative self-discipline prompted in part by the exhortations of watchful experts is the means of accomplishing this management.

Because sex is both the site of the literal production of bodies and a potent site for figuring self-discipline and control of one's individual body, it facilitates the mechanics of biopower. Sex is not just an accidental site of moral concern, a handy marker of moral standing in modernity where another marker might have done just as well. Sex works in particular ways within the modern regime of power. It works to produce modern individuals, both literally and subjectively. As a result, sex is a site for determining what is normal in modernity. This is why the moral health of an entire nation can be marked by whether a small minority of the population engages in particular sex acts, as the talk of American politicians makes clear.[6]

Biopolitics depends upon and manages contradiction: the autonomous individual does *not* exist autonomously, but is dependent for "his" life on others, most intimately other members of "his" household, but also the entire network of economic and political relations that sustain life. Biopolitics accounts for this relational dependence through the aggregation of the individual into populations that can be managed. Yet, while the concept of populations may appear to be horizontal aggregations of equal individuals, in actuality, the management of populations establishes hierarchies both within and between groups. This gathering up of persons into populations not only encourages life; it also breaks people down into different – and differentially treated – groups.

Both self-discipline and the control of populations are part of the apparatus of modern freedom, but this freedom is experienced differentially (Mbembe 2003; Puar 2007). Some populations manage themselves through the inducement to be normal. So, for example, the freedom of American mass culture is the freedom of individuals to choose, particularly through consumption, to be like everyone else. Other populations are actively controlled – for example, through the current emphasis on security measures that are organized along the lines of race, class, and citizenship. Just as normative discipline constitutes a particular, modern form of freedom, these networks of control are also in the service of freedom. In a security society, certain forms of social control ensure the freedom of the nation. Without such security, we are told, freedom would be threatened at every turn.

Sex is one of the central moral discourses that distinguish between a "free" and a "constrained" population (Lazreg 1988; Mohanty 1991). Moreover, sex is a site of the oscillation between freedom and control on which biopolitics depends. US public discourse is often understood as a battle between sexual regulation (often at the level of the state) and sexual licentiousness (often at the level of commerce or commercial culture).[7] A

Foucauldian analysis of biopower suggests, however, that the two sides of this argument represent the oscillation between outright control and the incitement to produce sexual freedom that marks the discourse of sexuality. Such oscillation continually recurs in US public life because the connection between freedom and control is obscured by the discourse of sexuality, just as the relations between different population groups are obscured by biopolitics. Advocates so often take up one side or the other rather than intervening in the dynamic itself due to the difficulty in the United States of acknowledging the ways that commercial freedoms depend upon government regulation. Moreover, with both the persistence of the demand to be sexual, which suffuses American culture with sexuality, *and* the sexually repressive policies of the US government, sex bears the burden of producing the modern ethical subject – one who produces a normal (meaning free and unrepressed) sexual self and whose sexual self is simultaneously well regulated and even controlled by the state. So, for example, the same members of the US government who have enforced sexual regulation may also inveigh against other societies for their sexual repression.

Christian Secularism

Placing the moral problematic of secular modernity at the centre of analysis shifts the usual understanding of why sex is so profoundly powerful in US public life, even as public discourse shifts ambivalently between overvaluation and undervaluation. It means that the problem for sexuality in the contemporary moment is not as much religion and the repression that religion supposedly entails as it is modern secularism and the biopolitics that allow for its embodiment.

Moreover, the secular is not so easily separated from the religious. As Ann Pellegrini and I have argued in *Secularisms* (2008), religion and secularism are best analyzed in relation to one another. Not only are religion and secularism mutually definitional – you know the meaning of one by its relation to the other – but the two terms are also historically interrelated, such that to understand the meaning of secularism in any part of the world, one must also understand the religion in relation to which a particular secularism may have developed. When thinking about the United States, we need to understand the specifically Christian version of secularism whose predominance ensures that Christian norms and values continue to frame the possibilities for US law, policy, and social life.

Specifically, in the United States secular approaches to sexuality are imbricated with a Protestant genealogy that connects sexuality to freedom as autonomy and to the market. As all religious studies scholars know, Max Weber (1930) identified the ways that the Protestant ethic was central to the formation of secular capitalism and the free market. Yet Weberian analysis does not draw attention to the fact that the Protestant Reformation also marked a major change in sexual relations, one that instituted a particular form of sexual freedom. Most important, the dominant strains of the Reformation tie the idea of individual freedom to the institution of marriage: the free individual is the individual whose sexual activity is regulated in marriage. This idea of freedom in marriage is also intimately entwined with the market. For Martin Luther (1961; see also Jakobsen 2005), and particularly for John Calvin (1960; see also Witte and Kingdon 2005), whose legacy has been extremely influential in the US context, the free individual is a householder whose freedom is expressed through the combination of the freedom to marry and the freedom to respond to God by doing the work of a calling.[8] Calvin's householder, whose freedom is maintained through self-discipline, prefigures the modern individual, whose autonomy is secured in the market. The role of self-discipline as the normative embodiment of a market society is explored extensively by Tracy Trothen in Chapter 8 of this volume. She shows, for example, how doping rules in elite sport, which allow certain enhancements while banning others, are used to create the impression that sporting contests are won only because of the athletes' self-disciplined activity, not because of any "unnatural" advantage.

This type of regulated activity becomes internal to a predominant meaning of secular, market-based American freedom even as it upholds religious genealogies of sexual regulation and freedom at different times, whether the Catholic counter-reformation (Taylor 2007) or the supposed Judeo-Christian ethic of the United States. As Jordan (2005) has documented, this overlap of the secular and religious has made a complex and contradictory genealogy of Christian (much less "religious") thought on sex and marriage appear to produce a singular and universal position on marriage in US law and policy. The autonomous individual who becomes the bearer of secular freedom is also the bearer of the discourse of sexuality, with its combined emphasis on regulation and incitement to liberation as well as its implication in the management of populations.

This Christian secular heritage thus informs the idea of freedom that is particularly powerful in US public life at the current moment, marked as it is by neoliberal globalization. One can argue that neoliberalism, with its emphasis on laissez-faire economics, has intensified both the discourse of freedom and that of the privatized individual. In other words, neoliberalism has intensified the components that contribute to the obsession with sexuality in the US public sphere. Freedom may be better than tolerance, but particularly in the context of neoliberalism, freedom may not be so free after all.

Alternative Visions of Freedom and Justice
If neoliberal economics is, in fact, dependent on sexual relations as the embodiment – the literal materialization – of market subjectivities, can nonheteronormative forms of sexuality provide the basis for alternative social formations? Certainly, sex alone will not carry the revolution. It is true that a number of social theorists have pursued the question of how sex can contribute to a more general project of economic emancipation, including Herbert Marcuse's (1955) idea of sexual liberation as a key to the end of exploitation, and Antonio Negri's (2005) idea that taking back our leisure time could be crucially subversive of capital. Given the regulatory nature of modern freedom, however, all of these strategies are both powerful and have the danger of promoting biopolitical control in the name of freedom. Here is where modern, Enlightenment values fall short and need reimagining.

The question is not just how to free sex from the bonds of both family and capital but also how to form relations, whether familial or not, that resist the logic of capital and in so doing open the door to alternative possibilities. Specifically, we need to consider forms of freedom and justice that are not based on the autonomous individual and thus do not require the self-discipline of biopower. Queering Enlightenment values opens possibilities because sex (queer and otherwise) is a site for the creation, enactment, and embodiment of different types of relationships. And these relationships form the basis for an alternative ethical vision.

To illustrate some of these possibilities, I now turn to a project co-sponsored by the Barnard Center for Research on Women and the community-based organization Queers for Economic Justice (QEJ). The project, called Desiring Change,[9] brings together activist groups connected by a commitment to the idea that "the best defence of new social possibility is the creation of a powerful alternative vision ... The project incorporates various perceptions of desire, gender, and sexuality into alliance and action, weaving them into the fabric of struggles to change the world" (Hollibaugh, Jakobsen, and Sameh 2009).

This vision is expansive and requires cross-issue organizing, so the Desiring Change project asks questions like: What are the specific connections between queer lives, queer desires, and social issues as diverse as adoption, poverty, immigration, alternative familial forms, homelessness, urban development, incarceration, and war? Just as the project hopes to connect desire to social change, I also hope to connect queer aspirations for freedom, albeit in a perverse form, to aspirations for social justice, including the economic justice that is the primary purview of QEJ.

Specifically, the project aspires to a new vision of the "general public," one that moves beyond tolerance and includes people who might understand themselves in opposition to each other, such as those who support families and the queers who are seen as the enemy of all that is familial. In other words, the exclusions, including the religious exclusions that are created through the current politics of sexuality, would not simply be reversed in this new vision, with queers and their allies now inside the public but religious conservatives now positioned as "other" and marginalized; rather, the point of the Desiring Change project is to develop a capacious vision of possibilities for public life. So, for example, in the context of the complex relations between conservative Hong Kong Canadian Christians and the multicultural Canadian public that Lee Wing Hin documents in Chapter 3 of this volume, Christian conservatives argue that the prospect of including same-sex marriage in Canadian public policy excludes Hong Kong Canadians because same-sex marriage violates their culture. Some versions of lesbian and gay politics might, in fact, be liable to this claim because they depend on a version of secularism that removes religion from public life. Alternatively, however, the queer public that Desiring Change imagines would be open to expressions of religious belief and to the ways that belief promotes political positions. Such a queer public would not, however, grant to religious belief a political trump card, any more than it would grant such status to the dominant norms of tolerance.

Such a view of the public means that not all conflicts are resolvable – some Christians and some queers may remain unreconciled – but the Desiring Change project also tries to find new ways of making substantive connections among groups that usually stand on opposite sides of the border defined by tolerance. Thus the vision of Desiring Change is to mobilize the feminist insight that desires and interests are not inherent in identities but are constituted through the ethics and politics of activity for social movement. The understanding of sexual ethics and its concomitant sexual politics in the United States was different as recently as the 1970s, when, for example, many churches in the Southern Baptist Convention were open on the ethical question of abortion because of their own commitment to norms of congregational autonomy and individual freedom. With the reconstitution of the Southern Baptist Convention throughout the 1980s, however, denominational control became the norm, and the politics of gender and sexuality shifted to the right. But these shifts are not definitive for all time, and evangelicals in the United States have begun to move again, this time away from a traditional focus on the family as the only means to a moral life. Openness to those who might become one's allies, even if such a relationship seems unlikely in any given political moment, is part of openness to the desire for change.[10]

As an example of how new ethical articulations can enable different relationships and alliances, consider the oft-invoked vulnerability of "families" in the midst of contemporary economic crises. "Family" is a word that has been used to narrow the boundaries of the public to include only those who live within certain norms, but if "families" are understood to be sites of freedom and justice, new connections among people become visible. Recurrent crisis is but the leading edge of economic shifts that have for the past several decades increased the vulnerability of working people, whatever their familial arrangements, in the United States and around the world. These shifts have included reductions in the provision of a social safety net as government services have been moved into the private sphere, with the result that only those with the individual means to pay might receive these services. The combination of reduced government services and an increased focus on for-profit corporations as the source of all social value is "neoliberal privatization" (Harvey 2007, 3). The vulnerabilities created by neoliberal privatization are potential sites for alliance, but they can also be exploited to divide groups. A clear articulation of the relational basis for social justice can help us to build a scaffolding of connection and to resist divisions among those whose interests and values might be actively aligned.

Perhaps most important for the Desiring Change project, the privatization that is the hallmark of a neoliberal system depends on services that are provided in the context of "private" relations, which are most often conceived of as familial. For example, healthcare practices have changed so as to shorten hospital stays and send people home to the care of their families as quickly as possible. Who provides the care that used to be provided by hospitals? The expectation is that "families" will do so.

The consequential burden on individuals and their relations can be extreme. People who can't afford to pay for care often have to quit their jobs in order to care for relations who are ill or injured. These burdens and attendant vulnerabilities are only increased for those who – for whatever reason – do not have a "family" to fall back on. Even if one has lived in a traditional family and remained married for a lifetime, the loss of a spouse may produce intense vulnerability, unless one's children can take on new responsibilities of care. But, for the people with whom Queers for Economic Justice works, the chances are low that such middle-class or wealthy relatives are able to help. And, with the full embrace of privatization, US society has said that these problems are the individual's to solve.

The Desiring Change project is not focused only on queer people, as the burdens of privatization can be intense for anyone – for the new mother who must leave the hospital and care for her infant child while still recovering herself, for the parents who must find schooling for their children when the public school system is underfunded and often unsafe, for the individuals who must choose between their jobs and caring for loved ones. Desiring Change is dedicated to making positive connections between these struggles and the lives of queer and transgendered people who have created nonfamilial systems of support.

And here we see the intersection between the broad system of neoliberal political economy and the personal desires and relations that are (thought to be) the appropriate subject of sexual politics. In particular, the labour done within the context of families is crucial to the neoliberal economic system as a whole. Individuals will have to find a way to endure these burdens themselves – privately. A neoliberal government has no concern for the bits and pieces of broken relationships; what matters is that some individuals be identified as personally responsible for the care of others. So, for example, many states require mothers to name the biological fathers of their children even if these men are abusive or simply not available. And the state government will pursue these men for child support, even if doing so delays the provision of any support for the child. Whether this child – or anyone – suffers is not the primary question in a neoliberal system; rather, the question is what individual will take responsibility.

Just as goods and services are privatized in this system, the negative consequences of the system are often felt in an intensely personal and private way, whether in the exhaustion of personally providing care that might be socially provided, the pain of broken relations that couldn't stand the strain, or the trauma of staying in an abusive relationship simply for the sake of survival. By taking these negative consequences seriously, however, we can set them in the light of alternative social possibilities. Queer people have developed such alternatives by building all kinds of relationships that meet both needs and desires. These creative responses provide another means of forging connections across issues since healthcare, economics, and sexuality, for example, all come together at the nexus of caring labour and so-called "private life."

The need to provide caring labour under conditions of vulnerability could be a point of connection between queer relationships and all kinds of families. Support for caring labour is needed in a variety of relationships, regardless of how they are defined. Recognizing and supporting people's range of values in building their relational lives has been termed "sexual democracy" (Duggan 2011-12). The basic ideals of democracy, freedom, and justice hold that people should be free to build lives under conditions of liberty and fairness and to pursue happiness as they define it. Yet this idea is rarely applied to sexuality or relational life, where prescriptive (and proscriptive) values often guide public policy.

There is, for example, a long history in the United States of denying relational recognition on the basis of race and ethnicity and then using accusations of sexual non-normativity as the basis for the denial of basic human rights and freedom. These practices have included the enslavement of African Americans and the refusal to recognize the marriages of slaves, laws against miscegenation and interracial marriage, the so-called 1965 "Moynihan report" on the crisis in the Black family, and the 1996 enactment of "welfare reform" (West 2000; Cott 2002; Chappell 2010). Similarly, with regard to immigrants to the United States, particularly non-Protestant immigrants of all races, a refusal to recognize familial relations has been the basis for exclusionary laws and discriminatory public policy (Fitzgerald 2006; Reddy 2011).

The democratic recognition of relationships also breaks the Christian (particularly the Calvinist) presumption of US public life. Opening the door to different kinds of "families" also opens the door to intimate relations that aren't ethically evaluated on the basis of their similarity to the Protestant family. One of the great worries articulated by those who do not understand religious diversity as a moral good, including academics like Samuel Huntington (2005) and Eric Kaufmann (2011), is that different religious communities embody "family values" that are not those of liberal Protestantism or secular humanism. In these narratives, those deeply devoted to religion are overly reproductive because of their religious beliefs, or they do not share a form of patriarchy with the dominant cultures of Europe and America and are thus less "free." Sexual democracy suggests that it is a mistake to invoke the liberal trick by denying freedom and equality to people because their relationships and their values are not those of the majority.

The intense and unpredictable relations of queer life that connect all kinds of people in all kinds of ways are incompatible with a model of tolerance that sets limits on the boundaries of acceptable difference, which are often determined by whether or not one's relational life can be fit into the dominant model of a "family."[11] But modern freedom will not in and of itself expand the boundaries of the public. If modern freedom is not to be the handmaiden of economic injustice, both freedom and justice must be reimagined beyond the bounds of sexual normativity. Sexual democracy imagines freedom and justice as open to a broad range of relational life. And this more dynamic model of public life can provide the basis for a holistic sexual ethics and politics that don't require us to remove either different people or different religions from our line of vision. This world – exciting, unexpected, and encompassing – is possible, but it will take both desire and change to make it a reality.

Notes

1 Even traditionally progressive and thus skeptical sites like the *Guardian* newspaper in London and the *Nation* weekly in New York heard Obama's Cairo speech as "a world away" from the approach of the Bush administration (Freedland 2009). The editor of the *Nation*, Katrina vanden Heuval (2009), simply called the Cairo speech "magnificent" in her blog. For a report that puts transnational interreligious relations definitively within the realm of national security, see Appleby and Cizik (2010). The press release for this report positions it as "the next step" after Obama's Cairo speech "in developing a strategy to engage religious communities of all faiths in addressing foreign policy challenges" (Chicago Council on Global Affairs 2010).
2 The controversy is briefly outlined by Banks 2011. For the current membership list see White House (2012).
3 For example, a 2006 CBS News poll found that 82 percent of Americans believed in God, that 9 percent believed in a "Universal Spirit," and that 8 percent did not believe in either (CBS News 2006). In contrast, a 2004 poll conducted by ICM Research for the British Broadcasting Corporation found that only 46 percent of respondents in the United Kingdom, 42 percent in Russia, and 28 percent in South Korea believed in God (BBC News 2004).
4 Interestingly, the phrase "and justice for all" occurs in the Pledge of Allegiance to the Flag (officially adopted by Congress in 1942), but it does not occur in either the Declaration of Independence or the US Constitution.
5 Both Bell (1985) and Bynum (1987) have argued convincingly that during the medieval period, food rather than sex was the primary site for the embodiment of morality and that the sin of greatest concern was gluttony rather than adultery, homosexuality, or other forms of sexual perversion. In the modern period, however, as food became more abundant in Europe and its consumption became less a matter of moral stricture, moral preoccupations shifted.
6 See, for example, Robert Byrd's speech on behalf of the Defense of Marriage Act in 1996. Byrd was a Democrat and not a member of the identified "religious right," yet when it came to the Defense of Marriage Act (legislation directly regarding sexuality), Byrd read from his family Bible on the floor of the Senate and then concluded, "Woe betide that society, Mr. President, that fails to honor that [Biblical] heritage and begins to blur that tradition which was laid down by the Creator in the beginning" (*Congressional Record*, S10110, 10 September 1996).
7 For an example of this kind of debate, in which the problem of sex in US public life is configured as either a regulatory Christian conservatism that produces state policy or a popular culture that promotes licentiousness, see Rosen's (2008) review of Dagmar Herzog's book on conservative Christian sexual culture, in which Rosen concludes that Herzog misses the point because the problem is not Christian conservatism but the licentiousness of teen sexual culture.

8 The foundational role of the Puritans in American culture establishes the place of the Calvinist heritage in mainstream American cultural and political life, although the implications and level of this influence are a matter of scholarly and public debate. On the scholarly debate, see Butler (1990) and Gaustad and Schmidt (2002). For the public debate as carried out on the Internet, see Jon Rowe's (2006) argument with Robert Ulrich (no date).
9 See http://bcrw.barnard.edu/publications/desiring-change.
10 For a full analysis of both the ethics and politics of alliance, see Jakobsen (1998).
11 For some consideration of how this sexual democracy might work in public policy, see DeFilippis et al. (2011-12).

References

Appleby, S., and R. Cizik. 2010. *Engaging Religious Communities Abroad: A New Imperative for U.S. Foreign Policy.* Report of the Taskforce on Religion and U.S. Foreign Policy. Submitted to the Chicago Council on Global Affairs. http://www.thechicagocouncil.org/Files/Studies_Publications/TaskForcesandStudies/Religion_2010.aspx.

Banks, A. 2011. Obama's Faith-Based Advisers: Round Two. 25 May. http://www.huffingtonpost.com/2011/02/07/obama-names-second-round-_n_819880.html.

BBC News. 2004. What the World Thinks of God. 26 February. http://news.bbc.co.uk/1/shared/spl/hi/programmes/wtwtgod/pdf/wtwtogod.pdf.

Bell, R.M. 1985. *Holy Anorexia.* Chicago: University of Chicago Press.

Berger, B.L. 2010. The Cultural Limits of Legal Tolerance. In *After Pluralism,* ed. P.E. Klassen and C. Bender, 98-126. New York: Columbia University Press.

Berlant, L., and L. Duggan. 2001. Introduction. In *Our Monica, Ourselves: The Clinton Affair and the National Interest,* ed. L. Berlant and L. Duggan, 1-8. New York: New York University Press.

Braunfeld v. Brown. 1961. 366 U.S. 599.

Butler, J. 1990. *Awash in a Sea of Faith: Christianizing the American People.* Cambridge, MA: Harvard University Press.

Bynum, C. Walker. 1987. *Holy Feast, Holy Fast: The Religious Significance of Food to Medieval Women.* Berkeley: University of California Press.

Calvin, J. 1960. *The Institutes of the Christian Religion.* Ed. J.T. McNeill. Trans. F.L. Battles. 2 vols. Philadelphia: Westminster.

CBS News. 2006. Poll. 6-9 April. http://www.pollingreport.com/religion.htm.

Chappell, M. 2010. *The War on Welfare: Family, Poverty, and Politics in Modern America.* Philadelphia: University of Pennsylvania Press.

Chicago Council on Global Affairs. 2010. Engaging Religious Communities Abroad: A New Imperative for U.S. Foreign Policy. Press release. http://www.thechicagocouncil.org/Files/Studies_Publications/TaskForcesandStudies/Religion_2010.aspx.

Congressional Record – Senate. 1996. Vol. 142, no. 123, Tuesday, 10 September.
Cott, N.F. 2002. *Public Vows: A History of Marriage and the Nation.* Cambridge, MA: Harvard University Press.
DeFilippis, J., L. Duggan, K. Farrow, and R. Kim, eds. 2011-12. *A New Queer Agenda.* Themed issue of *Scholar and Feminist Online* 10 (1-2), http://sfonline.barnard.edu/a-new-queer-agenda.
Duggan, L. 2000. *Sapphic Slashers: Sex, Violence, and American Modernity.* Durham, NC: Duke University Press.
–. 2004. *The Twilight of Equality: Neoliberalism, Cultural Politics and the Attack on Democracy.* Boston: Beacon.
–. 2011-12. After Neoliberalism? From Crisis to Organizing for Queer Economic Justice. In *A New Queer Agenda*, ed. J. DeFilippis, L. Duggan, K. Farrow, and R. Kim. Themed issue of *Scholar and Feminist Online* 10 (1-2), http://sfonline.barnard.edu/a-new-queer-agenda.
Emon, A.M. 2010. Pluralizing Religion: Islamic Law and the Anxiety of Reasoned Deliberation. In *After Pluralism: Reimagining Religious Engagement*, ed. C. Bender and P.E. Klassen, 59-81. New York: Columbia University Press.
Ferguson, R.A. 2003. *Aberrations in Black: Toward a Queer of Color Critique.* Minneapolis: University of Minnesota Press.
Fitzgerald, M. 2006. *Habits of Compassion: Irish Catholic Nuns and the Origins of New York's Welfare System, 1895-1920.* Champagne-Urbana: University of Illinois Press.
Foucault, M. 1980. *The History of Sexuality.* Vol. 1, *An Introduction.* Trans. R. Hurley. New York: Vintage.
–. 1991. Governmentality. In *The Foucault Effect: Studies in Governmentality*, ed. G. Burchell, C. Gordon, and P. Miller, 87-104. Chicago: University of Chicago Press.
Freedland, J. 2009. Barack Obama in Cairo: The Speech No Other President Could Make. 4 June. http://www.guardian.co.uk/world/2009/jun/04/barack-obama-speech-islam-west.
Gaustad, E., and L. Schmidt. 2002. *The Religious History of America: The Heart of the American Story from Colonial Times to the Present.* Rev. ed. New York: Harper Collins.
Goldman v. Weinberger. 1986. 475, U.S. 503.
Harvey, D. 2007. *A Brief History of Neoliberalism.* New York: Oxford University Press.
Hollibaugh, A., J.R. Jakobsen, and C. Sameh. 2009. Desiring Change. Report of the Barnard Center for Research on Women. http://bcrw.barnard.edu/wp-content/nfs/reports/NFS7-Desiring-Change.pdf.
Huntington, S.P. 2005. *Who Are We? The Challenges to America's National Identity.* New York: Simon and Schuster.
Jakobsen, J.R. 1998. *Working Alliances and the Politics of Difference: Diversity and Feminist Ethics.* Bloomington: Indiana University Press.
–. 2005. Sex + Freedom = Regulation: Why? *Social Text* 23 (3-4): 285-308.

—. 2010. Queer Relations: A Reading of Martha Nussbaum on Same-Sex Marriage. *Columbia Journal of Gender and Law* 19 (1): 133-78.
Jakobsen, J.R., and A. Pellegrini. 2003. *Love the Sin: Sexual Regulation and the Limits of Religious Tolerance.* New York: New York University Press.
—, eds. 2008. *Secularisms.* Durham, NC: Duke University Press.
Jordan, M. 2005. *Blessing Same-Sex Unions: The Perils of Queer Romance and the Confusions of Christian Marriage.* Chicago: University of Chicago Press.
Kaufmann, E. 2011. *Shall the Religious Inherit the Earth? Religion, Demography, and Politics in the Twenty-First Century.* London: Profile Books.
Kazanjian, D. 2003. *Colonizing Trick: National Culture and Imperial Citizenship in Early America.* Minneapolis: University of Minnesota Press.
Lazreg, M. 1988. Feminism and Difference: The Perils of Writing as a Woman on Women in Algeria. *Feminist Studies* 14 (1): 81-107.
Luther, M. 1961. *Martin Luther: Selections from His Writings.* Ed. and trans. J. Dillenberger. New York: Anchor Books.
Marcuse, H. 1955. *Eros and Civilization: A Philosophical Inquiry into Freud.* Boston: Beacon.
Mbembe, A. 2003. Necropolitics. Trans. L. Mientjes. *Public Culture* 15 (1): 11-40.
Mohanty, C.T. 1991. Under Western Eyes: Feminist Scholarship and Colonial Discourses. In *Third World Women and the Politics of Feminism,* ed. C.T. Mohanty, A. Russo, and L. Torres, 51-80. Bloomington: Indiana University Press.
Negri, A. 2005. *The Politics of Subversion: A Manifesto for the Twenty-First Century.* Boston: Polity.
Pierre-Pierre, G. 1997. Hasidic Community Opposes Bike Lane Plan. *New York Times,* 16 November. http://www.nytimes.com/1997/11/16/nyregion/hasidic-community-opposes-bike-lane-plan.html.
Puar, J.K. 2007. *Terrorist Assemblages: Homonationalism in Queer Times.* Durham, NC: Duke University Press.
Reddy, C. 2011. *Freedom with Violence: Race, Sexuality and the U.S. State.* Durham, NC: Duke University Press.
Rosen, H. 2008. In Bed with the Christian Right. *New York Times,* 31 August, BK16.
Rowe, J. 2006. One of the Worst Christian Nation Articles Yet. 15 May. http://jonrowe.blogspot.com/2006_05_01_archive.html.
Shah, N. 2005. Policing Privacy, Migrants, and the Limits of Freedom. *Social Text* 23 (3-4): 275-84.
Taylor, C. 2007. Sex and Christianity: How Has the Moral Landscape Changed? *Commonweal: A Review of Religion, Politics and Culture* 134 (16): 12-18.
Ulrich, R. n.d. Were the Founding Fathers Christian? http://www.libertyparkusafd.org/Madison/monographs%5CWere%20the%20Founding%20Fathers%20Christian.htm.

vanden Heuval, K. 2009. Obama: Reset and Refocus. 23 June. http://www.thenation.com/blog/obama-refocus-and-reset.

Weber, M. 1930. *The Protestant Ethic and the Spirit of Capitalism.* Trans. T. Parsons. New York: Charles Scribner's Sons.

West, T. 2000. The Policing of Poor Black Women's Sexual Reproduction. In *God Forbid: Religion and Sex in American Public Life,* ed. K.M. Sands, 135-54. New York: Oxford University Press.

White House. 2009. Obama Announces White House Office of Faith-Based and Neighborhood Partnerships. Press release. 5 February. http://www.whitehouse.gov/the_press_office/ObamaAnnouncesWhiteHouseOfficeofFaith-basedandNeighborhoodPartnerships.

–. 2012. About the President's Advisory Council on Faith-Based and Neighborhood Partnerships. http://www.whitehouse.gov/administration/eop/ofbnp/about/council.

Witte, J. Jr., and R.M. Kingdon. 2005. *Sex, Marriage, and Family in John Calvin's Geneva: Courtship, Engagement, and Marriage.* Grand Rapids, MI: William B. Eerdmans.

2

"Severely Normal"
SEXUALITY AND RELIGION IN ALBERTA'S BILL 44

Pamela Dickey Young

In June 2009 Alberta passed long-overdue human rights legislation – Bill 44: Human Rights, Citizenship and Multiculturalism Amendment Act – to include sexual orientation as a prohibited ground of discrimination. It had been directed to do so years before when its specific and intentional exclusion was challenged by Delwin Vriend et al. and found to be unconstitutional (see *Vriend* 1998).[1] However, in addition to finally including sexual orientation as one of the prohibited grounds of discrimination, Bill 44 also included provisions about education, more precisely about the right of parents to be informed when certain subjects were to be discussed in class. The passage reads as follows:

Notice to parent or guardian

11.1(1) A board as defined in the *School Act* shall provide notice to a parent or guardian of a student where courses of study, educational programs or instructional materials, or instruction or exercises, prescribed under that Act include subject-matter that *deals explicitly with religion, sexuality or sexual orientation*. (Government of Alberta 2009, emphasis added)

Bill 44 did not pass without notice. There were objections from a large number of sources, including human rights groups. The Alberta Teachers' Association, the Alberta School Boards Association, the Alberta School Councils' Association, and the College of Alberta School Superintendents released a joint statement on Bill 44 in June 2009. "These four groups, which often have divergent opinions and positions on specific educational issues, are solidly united in their view that the provisions in Bill 44 relating to education are unnecessary, unworkable and harmful to student learning. They are therefore calling on government to remove the offending provisions from the bill" (Alberta Teachers' Association 2009). Much of the press, both in Alberta and nationally, criticized and opposed Bill 44 (see Alberta Teachers' Association 2008-09; and Canadian Broadcasting Corporation 2009a). The Sheldon Chumir Foundation for Ethics in Leadership was particularly active in its opposition to the legislation. The foundation wrote opinion pieces and communicated directly with Lindsay Blackett, the minister of culture and community spirit, under whose auspices Bill 44 was introduced. It argued, among other things, that

> the proposed opt-out opens the door to all kinds of objections to the curriculum. It will have a chilling effect on classrooms and needlessly occupy teachers and administrators with providing advance notice about much of the curriculum rather than concentrating their time and resources on educating young Albertans for the knowledge economy and democratic citizenship.
>
> Bill 44 will impede the development of full critical thinking skills in Alberta's children and disrupt both the schools and the Human Rights Commission. (Keeping 2009, 6)

The Canadian province of Alberta is generally regarded as Canada's most politically and socially conservative province. It has consistently elected right-of-centre provincial governments since the 1930s. Alberta has a great variety of types of schools: publicly funded public schools, including faith-based schools; separate denominational schools, which are mostly Catholic schools; charter schools; francophone schools; one co-operatively federated school authority; and private but in part publicly funded schools (Hiemstra and Brink 2006; see also Government of Alberta 2010c).[2] However, Bill 44 does not actually apply to schools in this final category, which includes private religious schools, because they are privately governed.

Schooling in Alberta would seem to offer a wide market choice in terms of religion, where market choice means greater parental control over what is taught (Taylor 2001; Government of Alberta 2010c; see also Government of Alberta 2010a). School boards can offer alternative programs that, among other things, might be taught from the point of view of a particular religion.

School boards have introduced religious schools into the public system at various times. In 1999, for example, three formerly private Christian schools were admitted to the Edmonton public school system. Part of the argument for doing this went as follows:

> In addition, the district has learned though its Logos alternative program that non-denominational Christian education responds to a deeply felt need on the part of many families. Being able to serve the students of Edmonton Christian School would give the district the opportunity to earn the trust of families who have not previously been willing to entrust their children's education to the public system. (Edmonton Public Schools 1999, quoted in Taylor 2001, 31)

This statement is telling because it shows a desire to create public schools in response to the "deeply felt need" of the parents rather than according to a specific philosophy of education. In debates over funding religious schooling from the public purse, the rhetoric of choice is the one most often used – that parents should have choice – but the Logos schools[3] that entered the Edmonton Public School Board in 1999 relied much more on savvy lobbying efforts than they did on the popular views of parents (Taylor 2001). In comparison to dozens of Christian schools, some public and some private, there are not nearly as many schools related to other religious traditions, and most of these are private.[4]

There does not seem to have been huge pressure on the Alberta government to include provisions about schooling in Bill 44:

> There was something approaching zero public pressure for [Alberta premier Ed] Stelmach to strengthen parental rights at the school level. The strictest biblical believers have largely given up on the Godless public school system anyway, preferring to teach their kids at home, or entrusting them to the faithful arms of the Catholic board or the thriving sector of religious charter schools (one Calgary institution advertises

itself as a place where 'God is the principal'); everyone else seems to have been able to reach some amicable arrangement with their child's teacher, principal or school board using protections already afforded in the *School Act*. Filing this matter under the Human Rights Commission's mandate ensures that should something like this ever end up in court, it will be taxpayers now, not parents, who pick up the legal bills. (Libin 2009)

There were many questions about the specifics of the topics of instruction that the legislation would cover. For instance, the premier, Ed Stelmach, was quoted as saying that the bill was also meant to include teaching about evolution as among the things parents could object to (Audette 2009). But Lindsay Blackett reversed this position:

> This is opt-out on religious instruction not on grounds of religious beliefs. So the thought that somebody can get out of evolution using the fact that it's against their religious beliefs is not correct ... Evolution is not a part of religious studies, it's part of science curriculum, and there is nothing that will change that going forward. (Canadian Broadcasting Corporation 2009b)

Although Minister of Education Dave Hancock insisted that the bill didn't really change parental rights in Alberta since the School Act already allowed for parents to withdraw children if they objected to instruction about religion or sexuality, he requested a delay in the enactment of the legislation to allow more time for teachers and administrators to understand the full implications of the legislation. Although the bill was passed in 2009, it went into effect only in September 2010 after a changed version of the Alberta *Guide to Education* was prepared (Government of Alberta 2013).

The Alberta *Guide to Education* clarifies how Bill 44 will be applied in schools. The guide stresses that the requirements do not apply to "incidental or indirect references to religion, religious themes, human sexuality or sexual orientation" (Government of Alberta 2013, 16) and affirms that studying controversial issues is important in preparing students for life in Canadian society. It identifies a group of courses that deal "primarily and explicitly" with religion, human sexuality, and/or sexual orientation, but it also says that these are not the only courses that might be of concern. The guide goes to some lengths to say what "primarily and explicitly" means:

> For the instructional material, exercise, outcome or course to be considered to deal explicitly with religion, human sexuality or sexual orientation, there must be no question that the subject matter is *intended* to be about religion, human sexuality or sexual orientation. A religious interpretation of an otherwise non-religious subject matter would not be considered explicit. For example, the intent of including evolution in the science programs of study is to explore its foundation in scientific theory. Although there may be religious interpretations of the origin of life, the inclusion of evolution is not intended to be explicitly about religion. Similarly, in order to be considered explicitly about "human sexuality," an outcome, course, exercise or instructional material must also address human sexual behaviours. Therefore, outcomes within the science programs of study that deal only with the anatomy and physiology of human reproduction are not explicitly about human sexuality; however, outcomes in CALM [Career and Life Management] that examine aspects of healthy sexuality and responsible sexual behaviour are explicitly about human sexuality. (Ibid., 73-74, emphasis added)

Since Alberta allows faith-based education of a variety of sorts, all references to religion in faith-based education can be covered by a notice given to families on registration forms (ibid., 72-73).

But determining when a reference in the classroom is primarily and explicitly about "religion, sexuality or sexual orientation" could well prove over time to be a subjective matter. The bill has not been around long enough to know whether and how parents are going to mount challenges to what happens in school classrooms based on its provisions. By early 2013 no cases had yet come to the Alberta Human Rights Commission, but anecdotal evidence seemed to indicate that teachers had modified their teaching by avoiding certain topics so as not to be the subject of complaints (Steward 2012).

Discussion

This bill amending the Human Rights, Citizenship and Multiculturalism Act raises a number of interesting and important questions: (1) Why is this section contained in human rights legislation, not in legislation concerning schools? (2) Why is religion on the one hand put together with sexuality and sexual orientation on the other? (3) Which construals of sex and religion are abetted by the passage of Bill 44, and which ones are hindered?

Why Is This Section Contained in Human Rights Legislation, Not in Legislation Concerning Schools?

Given that this new section on education was placed in human rights legislation drafted to prohibit discrimination on the ground of sexual orientation, one suspects that, at least in the mind of the Alberta government, these opt-out clauses are in some way a response to this new inclusion. Because sexuality and sexual orientation are assumed to be such contentious issues for many people (here, Alberta voters), the inclusion of sexual orientation in human rights legislation apparently required a caveat that signalled to voters that this inclusion did not mean that the Government of Alberta had all of a sudden changed its mind on the matter of appropriate sexualities and begun to treat members of sexual minorities as normative citizens. Rob Anderson, Conservative member of the Legislative Assembly (MLA) for Airdrie-Chestermere, said, "There are thousands and thousands of parents, the silent majority, *severely normal* Albertans that are extremely happy with this legislation, that believe it's right to affirm the right of parents as being the primary educators of their children on these subjects" (Canadian Broadcasting Corporation 2009a, emphasis added). Religion is also a prohibited ground of discrimination in Alberta human rights legislation, but religion was included prior to the new clauses, so we might assume that it was the inclusion of "sexual orientation" that made Bill 44 necessary. That is, although religion is included in the legislation, religion is not itself the problem. The problem is when certain dominant and hegemonic religious views might be questioned if the whole matter of nonhegemonic and nondominant sexual orientations is raised.

In particular, the inclusion of a clause on schools in human rights legislation reflects one of the concerns that was raised all along the way, not just in Alberta but also in the Canadian context more broadly, by those who opposed the extension of rights to sexual minorities. The concern could be phrased in this way: if these rights were extended, schools would have to teach students that the family takes varying forms, including forms with gay and lesbian parents, and that homophobia is as problematic as racism. So schools are contested ground. Parents with convictions (religious or otherwise) that heterosexual pairing is the only normative form of relationship fear that their children might be taught otherwise. They do not want schools offering their children readings of sexuality that counter those they hear at home. So children can be removed from class if sexual orientation (or sexuality or religion) is the topic of discussion. This preys on a notion of children as vulnerable and needing protection from hearing certain things. The question of why the bill concerns these three specific topics, rather than others, will be discussed below.[5]

Parents in Alberta already had a fair amount of leeway in exempting children from instruction in school topics deemed controversial (see Government of Alberta 2010c, 50.2), so the placement of the clause in this human rights legislation is at least as much about sending a political signal that capitalizes on assumed voter fears over the vulnerability of children as it is about guaranteeing parental rights. Alberta's reluctance to pass human rights legislation protecting sexual minorities shows the government's fear that such legislation is politically unpalatable there. "Mr. Blackett told the *Globe and Mail* last spring that the parental rights provision was written into the bill as an olive branch to religious groups and conservative voters who might be offended by the move to recognize gay rights" (O'Neill 2009).

Another supposedly contentious area of teaching is "sexuality," which is not specifically mentioned elsewhere in the human rights legislation. To what, really, does "sexuality" refer? One might assume in this context that it does not refer to those "severely normal" parents whose heterosexual, procreative marriages provide the "norm" in "normal." So, as will be explored below, it is only particular construals of sexuality that are problematic.

Why Is Religion on the One Hand Put Together with Sexuality and Sexual Orientation on the Other?

Sex and religion are both topics to which a notion of privacy is often attached. Sex and religion are thought of by some – and often treated in Canada both in popular opinion and in judicial decision – as private matters.[6] As such, they are linked to the family as the primary vehicle for transmitting information and values. So the contention arises when these topics go public – when they are dealt with in schools, legislatures, and other public places. Perhaps these issues are even more contentious in

Alberta, which tends to be regarded as Canada's most conservative province both in terms of government and in terms of social mores.[7]

Public values are at play in making some things contentious but not others. Some views of religion and sexuality are more "equal" (that is, seen as more generally acceptable) than others. Here one often sees at work the cultural values of parental and other groups. Local school boards have some (but not total) latitude in determining what they approve for teaching. Most people want to see their own values at work – but these values may differ widely from place to place and from parent to parent. What values education should teach and why are contested questions.

Even though sex may be thought of as private, many parents have no concern with schools teaching (in public) about sexuality, sexual orientation, or religion as long as they teach the "proper" things; for example, heterosexuality and heterosexual pairings are not the subject of the controversy regarding sexual orientation and sexuality in the classroom. So sexuality is deemed a private matter only when it contradicts the hegemonic sexual norm. And conservative views of religion often bolster the notion of "proper" views of sexuality. Christianity is the culturally dominant religion in Canada. In terms of sheer statistics, the percentage of Albertans who claim to be Christian is slightly lower than the percentage of all Canadians who claim the same. According to the 2001 census (the most recent data on religion released by Statistics Canada), Alberta does not have as many Christians (only about 70%) as the Canadian average (about 76%). But Alberta also has a higher ratio of Protestants to Roman Catholics (about 39% versus 25.7%) than the national average (about 30% versus 43.2%). Further, more Albertans than all Canadians (6.9% versus 4.5%) claim to be some "other Christian" or "other Protestant" not accounted for in the more specific choices. The number of adherents of such churches as the Evangelical Missionary Church and the Christian and Missionary Alliance is also much higher in Alberta (1.4%) than in the rest of Canada (0.5%). And Alberta has a higher number of those who claim "no religion" (23.1%) than does Canada as a whole (16.2%) (Statistics Canada 2001). Below I speculate about how the religious makeup of Alberta might have made Bill 44 palatable to Albertans.

There is also no question about the cultural dominance of heterosexuality and about the construction of heterosexuality as normative. As Janet Jakobsen points out in Chapter 1 of this volume, sex is one of the ways used in North American society to determine what is "normal," and it therefore bears a huge moral weight. Despite the many court rulings to the contrary in Canada,[8] those who do not identify as heterosexual cannot assume that they will be treated by society, particularly by some religious forces in society, as equals.

Canadian discomfort with sexuality tends to stem from Canada's inheritance of Victorian values and, undoubtedly, from Canada's hegemonically Christian religious roots, whether Catholic or Protestant. Christians have, at least from the second century on, been both afraid of sex and often obsessed with it (Young 2011). Christianity has had an uneasy time trying to integrate views of sexuality with an ethos that prefers celibacy to marriage and that separates pure souls from bodies that have carnal appetites. Since the 1960s, Canadian society has come a long way in modifying its attitudes to sex. Nonetheless, not everyone is comfortable talking about sex. Further, there is a wide range of opinions and value sets related to what is thought to be "appropriate" sexuality. As a society, we have generally accepted that adults will live together before or instead of marrying. We have made huge progress on ensuring rights for sexual minorities. But we cannot assume that all Canadians agree with these moves.

Some Canadians are also uncomfortable talking about religion, although probably for different reasons than they avoid talking about sex. Canadians generally tend to think of themselves as living in a "secular" country, but about 76 percent of Canadians still claim to be Christians, as noted above, and 84 percent overall claim some religious affiliation (Statistics Canada 2001). That being said, most Canadians don't attend religious services regularly (Lindsay 2008). And, at least as reflected in places like the media, they tend not to want to think of themselves in the same way religiously as Americans think of themselves (e.g., Coggins 2008). In Canada the fact that Catholicism and Protestantism have both been important in relatively equal ways has meant in many parts of the country a dilution of the kind of Protestant individualism that seems to be important in the United States (Beaman 2005). Also, both in terms of sheer numbers and in terms of percentages, many fewer Canadians than Americans claim to be evangelicals (Reimer 2003).

Historically, religion has had a lot to say about sex – some religions more than others. Traditionally, Christianity has been sex-negative, and many forms of Christianity have developed a rules-based approach to sexuality, where to know what proper sexual conduct is, you just have to know the rules (e.g., De Rogatis 2005).

In Canada the default position on sexual orientation is heterosexuality. That is, most gays and lesbians and other sexual minorities do not find themselves represented in educational materials or discussions. James Chamberlain, a British Columbia teacher, asked that several children's books depicting families with gay and lesbian parents be included as supplementary in the province's K-1 curriculum. The Surrey School Board, primarily on the basis of the religious objections of some parents, declined to do this. The case finally came to the Supreme Court of Canada (*Chamberlain* 2002), which pushed the decision back to the school board but also said that the board had violated the principles of secularism and tolerance adhered to in BC schools by taking parents' religious objections to be central.

In the case of Alberta, the prohibited discussions of sexual orientation presumably include any that have the potential to challenge normative heterosexuality. What message is being sent if, any time the whole question of nonheterosexuality might possibly come up, parental permission is needed for students to take part in the discussion?

For some people, any talk about sexuality – which, according to the legislation, seems not to include sexual orientation since it has to be specifically singled out – is threatening if the assumed "rules" about sexuality are questioned. One of the operative theories in opposition to sex education is that any information about sex leads to sexual activity. One sees this, for example, in the view of some evangelical Christians that sex should be prohibited until marriage, after which sex is supposed to be wonderful with the right partner – sexuality is a valve you keep turned off until you turn it on full blast at marriage (De Rogatis 2005, 109). For evangelical Christians, the lack of sex education means that those who do not or cannot adhere to the strict rules about sexuality are less likely to have contracepted sex when they do have sex before marriage (Regnerus 2007, 140-47).

People often confuse teaching about religion with indoctrination and teaching about sexuality with advocacy for "alternative" lifestyles. This is found on both ends of the religious spectrum – among those who are wary of all religion and among those who think there is only one legitimate religious way. For members of this latter group, there is the fear that teaching about a variety of religious paths might seem to suggest that their way is not the "right" way. Those who think that religion can be fanatical and problematic often worry that any and all teaching about religion will try to convince others of the exclusive merits of a particular religious way.

Although some liberal parents do not want any "religion" taught to their children, and might therefore be happy to be able to challenge the teaching of religion in schools, Bill 44 was primarily intended not to take such views into account but to support the views of more conservative Christians (see Trottier 2012), as will be argued below.

Canadians do not, for the most part, like overt religious talk from their politicians. And Canadian policies on multiculturalism imagine the nation as welcoming all religious traditions as well as other sorts of diversity. Many Canadians do not want one kind of conservative Christian politics to dominate the landscape. But the alternative is not to ignore religion. It might be useful to know about a politician's religious conviction (or lack thereof) because it is one important clue to how he or she might view the world and make decisions.

Determining what mentions of sexuality, sexual orientation, and religion count as appropriate subjects for teaching is certainly a matter of worry for school teachers and administrators. There are already protocols for dealing with sensitive subjects, and they require using these topics to conduct exploration, not to communicate a single point of view (see Government of Alberta 2013, 16). When is teaching about any of the above related to science, and when is it not? If evolution is not about religion because it is taught in science class (although some religious parents might be offended), could teaching about, say, the science behind various birth control methods or the avoidance of HIV be the same? Could teaching about the Bible (or the Qur'an or the Vedas) as literature be part of a language class?

There is no inherent reason why sexuality, sexual orientation, and religion should be lumped together. However, the special naming of sexual orientation in Bill 44 does pinpoint what the Alberta government assumes will be discomfort with certain (but not all) sexual orientations. Further, placing Bill 44 in the cultural context of Alberta helps us to see that sex, sexual orientation, and religion are lumped together here as a means to support the twin cultural hegemonies of conservative Christianity and heterosexual pairing.

Which Construals of Sex and Religion Are Abetted by the Passage of Bill 44, and Which Ones Are Hindered?

What problem was Bill 44 meant to solve? Alberta dragged its heels for eleven years after it was directed by the Supreme Court to amend its Human Rights Act to prohibit discrimination on the grounds of sexual orientation. Despite government officials' protests to the contrary, there must have been some reason that it took so long for this to happen.[9] Of course, given the lively discussion on Bill 44, one cannot assume that such an amendment would be unpalatable to all Albertans, but the Conservative Party in Alberta (the province's "natural ruling party") must have thought that it would be a political minefield to raise the issue of equal rights for sexual minorities. This notion is affirmed in Lindsay Blackett's comment to the *Globe and Mail*, quoted above, that Bill 44 was framed as it was to be an "olive branch" to religious people and Conservative voters. Thus Bill 44 was meant to solve not a problem of education or human rights but a problem of politics. The government tried to serve up the unpalatable in a way that would be palatable to those it considered its primary constituency.

That Bill 44 was framed by Blackett, a minister of the government, so as not to offend religious people is an important clue to the way that sexuality, sexual orientation, and religion are to be understood in this discourse. Specifically, sexuality and sexual orientation are meant to be read as problematic. Presumably, there are unproblematic sexualities and unproblematic sexual orientations. Those "severely normal" parents evoked by Conservative MLA Rob Anderson have probably all had sex lives. But the Alberta government presumes that their sexuality is, by implication, "normal" sexuality. One can speculate that if all teaching about sexuality encouraged premarital abstinence and advocated sex only within heterosexual marriage that "sexuality" would raise very few problems, certainly not problems whose discussion would require parental permission. Thus the problem is not "sexuality" but understandings of sexuality that are broader than the assumed Conservative voter's norm. The legislation enforces an understanding of sexuality that is strongly connected to the official understanding of sexuality held by evangelical Christians and Roman Catholic Christians as well as by conservative members of other religious traditions.

Likewise, if all discussions of sexual orientation assumed heteronormativity as the good and rightful position, such discussions would not generally be a threat. Although one can see the possibility of some parents wanting their children to be exposed to a wide variety of understandings of sexuality and sexual orientation, these do not seem to be the parents whom the Alberta Government had in view in the writing of Bill 44. Evangelical Protestants and Roman Catholics hold official views that disapprove of "homosexuality." Beyond Blackett's affirmation that this bill does have, in part, to do with the religious views of some parents, one can also speculate about the connection between Bill 44 and conservative Christianity by extrapolation from the same-sex marriage debate in Canada, where virtually the entire opposition to same-sex marriage came from religious sources and where the preponderance of these sources were Christian (Young 2010). There do not seem to be any organized forums for religious "nones" in Canada, and even if there were, it appears unlikely, based on the example of the same-sex marriage debate, that they would set themselves up to support the measure that Bill 44 enshrines. The problem posed by sexual orientation is that its discussion might threaten the heterosexual norm or might raise the possibility that there are socially approved sexual orientations beyond heterosexuality. Again, we can extrapolate from the debate over same-sex marriage, where conservative Christians argued that if same-sex marriage was legalized, their children might be taught in school that same-sex relationships were legitimate and appropriate (see Young 2006, 2010).

Here, the sexuality and sexual orientations that are diminished in their legitimacy are those that do not conform to the dominant norm. An observer can hardly be blamed for assuming that, based on Bill 44, sexual minority students and even those who have premarital heterosexual sex might come to an understanding that their sexual lives are less approved of, less "normal," than those of others because their sexual lives cannot even be discussed in class without parental permission.

What kind of religion is held out for approval here, and what sort is seen to be more questionable? At first glance, it might seem that religious pluralism in Alberta is affirmed by this legislation because it appears to take seriously the religious choices of parents. There are a lot of options in Alberta for religious schooling that is either fully or partially funded by the public, and the importance of parental choice about schooling, especially religious schooling, is one of the central themes that Taylor (2001) discovered in her longitudinal study of Alberta schools. But Bill 44 was not conceived with the intent of safeguarding just any kind of religion or all kinds of religion. Since all discussions of "religion" are singled out as problematic, Bill 44 appears to be neutral on religion. However, questions can be asked about discussions of religion and the problems associated with them that interrogate just how neutral the bill really is. One possible construal would read discussions of "religion" in the classroom as the opposite of discussions of sexuality and sexual orientation. That is, the parents who might not want sexuality discussed might be parents who would welcome the discussion of religion and vice versa. So the high percentage of parents in Alberta who claim no religion (noted above) might be wary of schools teaching about religion. It is certainly possible, given the preponderance of religious schools in Alberta, that such parents would worry that all talk about religion would be instruction in a particular religion, especially given that in Alberta school boards can and do prescribe religious instruction and religious exercises for students (Government of Alberta 2010c, 50.1). But it is precisely this prescription that leads to the conclusion that it is not the nonreligious parents who are the main concern of Bill 44. Rather, the conclusion drawn here from the overall situation of religion in Alberta schools is that Bill 44 caters to religious conservatives who do not want their children exposed to teaching that presents a wide variety of religious traditions as equally valid. This conclusion is again reinforced by Blackett's comment that the bill was aimed at religious parents. Although there are some non-Christian religious schools in Alberta, the vast majority of religious schools are Christian, either Roman Catholic or conservative Protestant. In these (and other religious) schools, "religion" can be discussed because parents' religious leanings are disclosed when they register their children; and when parents send their children to these schools, they agree to the teaching of religion from the school's religious perspective. In other schools, discussion of religion in class might lead to the assumption that no particular religion has a monopoly on truth, thus upsetting parents who want to be in control of the kind of religion their children are taught (Government of Alberta 2013, 16). But rather than making parents responsible for religious education, which would eliminate the idea that schools are responsible for teaching students how to be religious in particular ways, the school system in Alberta has positioned itself as a parental proxy in this regard by relying on parents to object under Bill 44 when teaching about religion does not adhere to their particular views. As Janet Jakobsen points out in Chapter 1 of this volume, the version of secularism that Americans (here North Americans) have adopted is a "Christian" version of secularism, one that supports heteronormativity even while it claims not to be influenced unduly by Christian values.

The Government of Alberta fosters religious pluralism in schools insofar as those with enough voice and enough lobbying power can either develop their own religious schools or influence the discussions in other classrooms. But the religious diversity being fostered is religious diversity within a narrow range of choices. First, it is hegemonically Christian and, within Alberta, largely Protestant Christian (for discussions of Christian hegemony within Canada, see Beaman 2005; and O'Toole 2000). Second, it would seem to favour those voices who encourage conservative responses to religion – that is, those voices whose worries about religion are clear and authoritative and who see and teach religion as a set of given rules to which one must adhere – for it is these voices who are most disturbed by "discussions" of religion.

Nonetheless, on the face of it, religious diversity is presented as a good thing insofar as Alberta has decided to allow for a wide variety of religious schooling under the public purse (notwithstanding that most of the religious schooling that it funds is Christian schooling). If religious diversity is good, why is sexual diversity not? If, as the Government of Alberta assumes, Albertans are happy with a wide variety of religious choices, why does the idea of choice not extend to sexual diversity? As far as I can tell, there are no Alberta schools directed toward the sexual minority population. Although the Alberta Teachers' Association has published a teachers' guide to *Gay-Straight Student Alliances in Alberta Schools* (Alberta Teachers' Association and Wells 2006), there is no mention of this guide on the Alberta Education website. Alberta Education has a policy on "Diversity in shared values," where diversity is understood in the following terms: "Education programs and instructional materials referred to in subsection (1) must not promote or foster doctrines of racial or ethnic superiority or persecution, religious intolerance or persecution, social change through violent action or disobedience of laws" (Government of Alberta 2010, 3.2). This policy further underlines the idea that only some kinds of diversity should be promoted in Alberta schools. Although religious intolerance is clearly mentioned, there is nothing parallel about intolerance of those of diverse sexualities or sexual orientations. In the

Alberta case, Christian hegemony seems alive and well, and homonormativity seems a somewhat distant dream.

Thus protection of a certain way of being religious would seem to militate against any recognition of "polymorphous" sexuality (Gudorf 2001, 884). Jakobsen and Pellegrini (2003, 103-26) regard this situation in the United States as limiting the "free exercise of sex" while fostering the "free exercise of religion." In the Canadian Charter of Rights and Freedoms, although both sexual orientation and religion are now prohibited grounds of discrimination, religion is also enshrined in Section 2 as a fundamental freedom. If we extend the Jakobsen and Pellegrini idea to the Canadian context, we might ask for a parallel freedom of sexual identity and expression. Freedom of religion has historically been limited when it is judged to come into clash with other fundamental freedoms. The same holds true for freedom of sexual identity and expression. That people might have a difficult time understanding why freedom of sexual identity and expression is necessary seems to echo in the Canadian context what Jakobsen and Pellegrini (ibid., 19) find in the United States, namely that sex is "inherently 'trouble.'" And this observation is true in spite of Canada's guarantees that one cannot discriminate on the basis of sex or sexual orientation, for nondiscrimination, important as it is, is a negatively stated right. There are no positively stated sexual rights in the Charter, except those that might be more generally stated in Section 2b in terms of freedom of opinion and expression. Maybe there is room for a notion of "multi-sexualism" or sexual pluralism that does not use tolerance as its main concept. In the same way that we need to move beyond "tolerance" as the main way to treat religious diversity, we need to move beyond "tolerance" as the main way to treat sexual diversity (see Jakobsen, Chapter 1, this volume).

Beaman (2011, 452-55) discusses what she calls "deep equality" as a strategy for managing religious diversity, which provides an alternative to the use of tolerance and reasonable accommodation. According to Beaman, deep "equality does not mean sameness." It begins from a "position of shared humanity" and requires an approach of "humility." For Beaman, some of the factors that need to be addressed in seeking deep equality are the colonial postcolonial context, a willingness of the courts to reshape existing legal boundaries, a "meaningful" valuing of the multicultural character of Canada, and a language that begins with the "equality of members of religious minorities."

In examining whether a complainant should have been required to remove her niqab when giving evidence in the Ontario Superior Court, Beaman squarely focuses on religious minorities. For religious minorities, the legacy of colonialism and its attendant racism are central factors to be interrogated. And multiculturalism must be embraced, not just given lip service. In the case of Bill 44, the contours of deep equality may need to be drawn somewhat differently. First, although colonialism might well come into play insofar as the multiplication of Alberta religious schools does serve a few religious minorities, it was not colonialism but Christian hegemonies that were the pervasive force in the promulgation of Bill 44. In this case, one needs to critically examine hegemonic forces, religious or otherwise, in order to see where and how these are being employed in the guise of neutrality. Second, to foster pluralism, we need to rethink the boundaries that mark out and divide those who are normative sexually from those who are not, as well as those who are normative religiously from those who are not. Canadian law has gone some way in questioning and reshaping these boundaries for sexual minorities, but as the Alberta bill makes clear, these gains are not as deeply entrenched as one might hope. Deep equality requires that we make space for a wide variety of voices and positions to be heard – and not just heard but also seriously considered. This means hearing religious minorities, who were curiously silent in this debate, and sexual minorities. Third, deep equality does not require that one forgo all judgment about various positions, but it does require that the criteria for judgments be clear and transparent. Some members of religious minorities might have difficulties with some members of sexual minorities and vice versa. (And, of course, some members of religious minorities are also members or supporters of sexual minorities.) The case study of Bill 44 shows that any "deep equality" vis-à-vis religion, including minority religion, also requires a notion of "deep equality" vis-à-vis sexuality. That is, because some forms of religion have such strong views of appropriate sexualities and sexual mores, religious groups also have to critique their own hegemonies. Thus deep equality requires an expansive capacity for self-critique of the ways that one's own normative assumptions limit the humanity of others – whether because of their religious identities, their sexual identities, or both. In Alberta the "problem" of religion is dealt with by funding multiple sorts of religious schools. But such a strategy does not even begin to take account of how this approach might reinforce certain religious and sexual hegemonies rather than call them into question. Surely, one does not have to dispossess sexual minorities to speak of religious minorities and vice versa.

Because "deep equality" requires an assumption of shared humanity and a position of humility, members of sexual or religious minorities, and members of both, have to bring assumptions of shared humanity and a position of humility to their dealings. Unless we move beyond the idea that we have to decide who is the more discriminated against, it will be difficult to move toward affirmations of human dignity for all (see Moreau 2006; and Réaume 2006).

In Bill 44 the Alberta government has taken an ambiguous approach to the question of whether religion, sexuality, and sexual orientation are public or private matters. On the one hand, the control over such matters is largely placed in parental hands, which shows that both religion and sexuality are understood as belonging primarily in the sphere of the family and that entrenching the family's views and values is more important than exposing children to a broader range of views and values.

Understanding religion and sexuality as private matters has social costs. Relegating them to the private sphere means that public critique or examination of either becomes difficult. Absent public critique or examination of religion and sexuality, one is left with the impression that what one believes or does in private is of no public concern. This has had different effects on religion and on sexuality. In the matter of religion, it has meant that religion is considered a matter of private belief and practice. If private, there are no real grounds for critique: everyone's religiosity is as valid or invalid as anyone else's. But further, if private, any manifestation of religion in the public sphere is often viewed with suspicion, as though it has no right to be there at all.

If sexuality and sexual orientation are viewed as private, one parallel with religion is that any (non-normative) sexuality that seeks the public gaze is often deemed problematic, as in, "I don't care what those people do in private, but don't expose me or my children to it." But further, if sexuality and sexual orientation are deemed private, the hegemonies of married heterosexual sexuality are never really challenged.

The Government of Alberta has taken a stance that religion does belong in public schooling in certain ways, and it funds many of these ways. Some courses that include sexuality are also funded in Alberta but not nearly in the comprehensive way that religion is funded. So religion is a public matter in Alberta insofar as the public purse extensively supports certain ways of being religious. In Alberta, however, a decision has been made that, apart from making the schools conform to curricular standards (and there are even some variances here), the schools can teach more or less what they please in relation to religion, which amounts to treating religion as a private matter.

Although Bill 44 purports to regulate both sexuality and religion, it seems that the bill regulates certain kinds of sexuality and certain kinds of religion by privileging other understandings of sexuality and other kinds of religion. The de facto established religion in Alberta (more Protestant than Catholic but partaking of both) creates and maintains the de facto established sexuality of Alberta: married, heterosexual monogamy.

Notes

1 Sexual orientation was read into the Canadian Charter of Rights and Freedoms as a prohibited ground of discrimination in 1995. Also, the *Vriend* case is another where sex, politics, and religion collide because Vriend was fired from a postsecondary religious institution, the King's College in Edmonton, because he was gay.
2 An article in the *Globe and Mail* (Hammer, 2011) details parental objections in Morinville, Alberta, to the fact that the only *public* school board in Morinville is a Catholic school board, the Greater St. Albert Catholic Regional Division.
3 The Logos Education Society was formed in 1977 to lobby the Calgary Board of Education to provide nondenominational Christian schools. Public funding was provided by the Calgary board for a few years and then discontinued. Private Logos schools continued to open and continued to lobby for public funding from various Alberta school boards. In 1999 Edmonton decided to fund these schools as public schools. In efforts to lobby the Edmonton Public School Board, the chief figures for Logos were not parents but a retired school principal and three retired professors of education. For a fuller history, see Taylor (2001).
4 A quick count revealed five Jewish schools, three Islamic schools, and two Sikh schools in Alberta.
5 For views on how schools are contested sites of power, see Shipley (Chapter 4, this volume) and the discussion of *Chamberlain v. Surrey School District No. 36* (2002) below.

6 See, for example, *Syndicat Northcrest v. Amselem* (2004), where the Supreme Court of Canada treats religion as very much a matter of private practice.
7 See, for example, Flanagan (2010).
8 See, for example, *Haig and Birch v. Canada* (1992), *Egan v. Canada* (1995), and *M. v. H.* (1999), which together established far-reaching rights for sexual minority persons.
9 Audette (2010) quotes Minster Lindsay Blackett as saying, "I think that as a government we're more open, accessible and aware of issues with regard to sexual orientation ... I think we show that we're tolerant and accessible and we'll take the lead any time those groups are actually attacked, but we haven't had any issues like that. I think Albertans are much more tolerant than we give them credit for. I think there was a lot of hue and cry over what would happen and I don't think anybody's seen that happen. I think it will die down and we'll move forward and we'll be a better province for it."

References

Alberta Teachers' Association. 2008-09. The Media on Bill 44. *ATA News* 43 (18). http://www.teachers.ab.ca/Publications/ATA%20News/Volume%2043/Number18/SpecialFeatureonBill44/Pages/ThemediaonBill44.aspx.

–. 2009. Submission to the Premier of Alberta: Regarding Bill 44, *Human Rights, Citizenship and Multiculturalism Amendment Act*. 8 May.

Alberta Teachers' Association and K. Wells. 2006. *Gay-Straight Student Alliances in Alberta Schools: A Guide for Teachers*. http://www.teachers.ab.ca/SiteCollectionDocuments/ATA/Publications/Human-Rights-Issues/Gay%E2%80%93Straight%20Student%20Alliances%20in%20Alberta%20Schools%20A%20Guide%20for%20Teachers.pdf.

Audette, T. 2009. Opponents Step Up Attacks on Human Rights Bill; Parental Rights Law a "Slippery Slope," Says Ethics Group. *Edmonton Journal*, 5 May.

–. 2010. Bill 44: One Year Later. *Edmonton Journal*, 31 May.

Beaman, L. 2005. The Myth of Pluralism, Diversity, and Vigor: The Constitutional Privilege of Protestantism in the United States and Canada. *Journal for the Scientific Study of Religion* 42 (3): 311-25.

–. 2011. "It was all slightly unreal": What's Wrong with Tolerance and Accommodation in the Adjudication of Religious Freedom? *Canadian Journal of Women and Law* 23 (2): 442-63.

Canadian Broadcasting Corporation. 2009a. Alberta Passes Law Allowing Parents to Pull Kids Out of Class. 2 June. http://www.cbc.ca/news/canada/story/2009/06/02/alberta-human-rights-school-gay-education-law.html.

–. 2009b. Proposed Alberta Law Doesn't Make Evolution Classes Optional: Minister. 4 May. http://www.cbc.ca/technology/story/2009/05/04/cgy-evolution-alberta-human-rights.html.

Chamberlain v. Surrey School District No. 36. 2002. 4 R.C.S. 710, 2002 CSC 86.

Coggins, J. 2008. Comment: American Religious Landscape May Be Changing. 13 March. http://canadianchristianity.com/nationalupdates/2008/080313comment.html.

De Rogatis, A. 2005. What Would Jesus Do? Sexuality and Salvation in Protestant Evangelical Sex Manuals, 1950s to the Present. *Church History* 74 (1): 97-137.

Edmonton Public Schools. 1999. Recommendation from Superintendent re: Edmonton Christian Schools Alternative Programs. 25 May.

Egan v. Canada. 1995. 2 S.C.R. 513.

Flanagan, T. 2010. Alberta's One Shot Wonder. *Globe and Mail,* 25 May.

Government of Alberta. 2009. *Bill 44: Human Rights, Citizenship and Multiculturalism Amendment Act.* http://www.assembly.ab.ca/ISYS/LADDAR_files/docs/bills/bill/legislature_27/session_2/20090210_bill-044.pdf.

–. 2010a. *Inspiring Education: Alberta's Vision for Education.* http://education.alberta.ca/department/ipr/inspiringeducation.aspx.

–. 2010b. Opportunities for Choice in Education. http://education.alberta.ca/parents/educationsys/ourstudents/iv.aspx.

–. 2010c. *School Act.* http://www.qp.alberta.ca/574.cfm?page=s03.cfm&leg_type=Acts&isbncln=9780779733941.

–. 2013. *Guide to Education: ECS to Grade 12.* http://education.alberta.ca/media/7570773/guidetoed2013.pdf.

Gudorf, C. 2001. The Erosion of Sexual Dimorphism: Challenges to Religion and Religious Ethics. *Journal of the American Academy of Religion* 69 (4): 863-91.

Haig and Birch v. Canada. 1992. Court of Appeal for Ontario, 9 O.R. (3d) 495 (C.A.).

Hammer, K. 2011. In an Alberta Town, Parents Fight for a Secular Education. *Globe and Mail,* 4 March, A23.

Hiemstra, J., and R.A. Brink. 2006. Advent of a Public Pluriformity Model: Faith-Based School Choice in Alberta. *Canadian Journal of Education* 29 (4): 1157-91.

Jakobsen, J.R., and A. Pellegrini. 2003. *Love the Sin: Sexual Regulation and the Limits of Religious Tolerance.* Boston: Beacon.

Keeping, J. 2009. Letter to Lindsay Blackett. 8 May. http://www.chumirethicsfoundation.ca/files/pdf/Letter%20to%20Min%20Blackett_Bill_44_050809.pdf.

Libin, K. 2009. Ed Stelmach, Up to His Knees in Turd. *National Post,* 6 May.

Lindsay, C. 2008. Canadians Attend Weekly Religious Services Less Than 20 Years Ago. *Matter of Fact* (3): 1-3. http://www.statcan.gc.ca/pub/89-630-x/2008001/article/10650-eng.pdf.

M. v. H. 1999. 2 S.C.R. 3.

Moreau, S. Reibetanz. 2006. Equality Rights and the Relevance of Comparator Groups. *Journal of Law and Equality* 5 (1): 81-96.

O'Neill, K. 2009. Education Minister Wants Alberta Parents' Rights Law Delayed. *Globe and Mail,* 27 August.

O'Toole, Roger. 2000. Canadian Religion: Heritage and Project. In *Rethinking Church, State, and Modernity: Canada Between Europe and America*, ed. David Lyon and Marguerite Van Die, 34-51. Montreal and Kingston: McGill-Queen's University Press.

Réaume, D. 2006. Law v. Canada (Minister of Employment and Immigration). *Canadian Journal of Women and the Law* 18 (1): 143-88.

Regnerus, M. 2007. *Forbidden Fruit: Sex and Religion in the Lives of American Teenagers*. New York: Oxford University Press.

Reimer, S. 2003. *Evangelicals and the Continental Divide: The Conservative Protestant Subculture in Canada and the United States*. Montreal and Kingston: McGill-Queen's University Press.

Statistics Canada. 2001. Selected Religions, for Canada, Provinces and Territories – 20% Sample Data. http://www12.statcan.ca/english/census01/products/highlight/religion/Page.cfm?Lang=E&Geo=PR&View=1a&Code=01&Table=1&StartRec=1&Sort=2&B1=01&B2=All.

Steward, G. 2012. Big Chill Hits Alberta Classrooms. *Toronto Star,* 10 September.

Syndicat Northcrest v. Amselem. 2004. 2 S.C.R. 551.

Taylor, A. 2001. "Fellow Travellers" and "True Believers": A Case Study of Religion and Politics in Alberta Schools. *Journal of Education Policy* 16 (1): 15-37.

Trottier, J. 2012. Alberta Refuses to Give Parents Freedom from Religion in Schools. *National Post,* 15 February. http://life.nationalpost.com/2012/02/15/justin-trottier-alberta-parents-given-no-freedom-from-religion-in-schools.

Young, P. Dickey. 2006. Same-Sex Marriage and Christian Churches in Canada. *Studies in Religion/Sciences Religieuses* 35 (1): 3-23.

–. 2010. Taking Account of Religion in Canada: The Debates over Gay and Lesbian Marriage. *Studies in Religion/Sciences Religieuses* 39 (3): 333-61.

–. 2011. It's All about Sex: The Roots of Opposition to Gay and Lesbian Marriages in Some Christian Churches. In *Faith, Politics and Sexual Diversity in Canada and the United States,* ed. D. Rayside and C. Wilcox, 165-76. Vancouver: UBC Press.

3

"I'm Not Homophobic, I'm Chinese"
HONG KONG CANADIAN CHRISTIANS AND THE CAMPAIGN AGAINST SAME-SEX MARRIAGE

Lee Wing Hin

As Chinese Canadians, in Chinese culture, we define marriage as being between two different genders, and we believe our culture should be honoured in this multicultural society.

> – Katherine Yu, statement at a meeting of the Standing Committee on Justice and Human Rights, 11 April 2003[1]

Marriage as the union of male and female runs so deep in the Chinese collective psyche that it is the foundation of culture and civilization ... For us the redefinition of marriage amounts to taking away from us a part of our being, a part of our culture ... Many feel betrayed that this significant aspect of Chinese culture is not being respected, even in a country that continues to preach multiculturalism and pluralism ... They want to stop what they perceive to be a forced colonization of their cultural life world.

> – Reverend Dominic Tse, statement at a meeting of the Legislative Committee, 18 May 2005

The excerpts above highlight the two central messages in Hong Kong Canadian public statements against the legalization of same-sex marriage during the heated debates that took place in Canada from 2002 to 2005. Campaigners emphasized that Chinese cultures and peoples universally condemn homosexuality and same-sex unions. In addition, they argued that Hong Kong Canadian voices must be heard in Canadian social and political arenas since Canada's multiculturalism policies mandate the inclusion of all cultural views. On these bases, they insisted that their belief in "traditional marriage" must be upheld and that the proposal for same-sex marriage must be rejected. However, Chinese texts and interviews I conducted reveal that the public insistence on Chinese cultural "traditions" of cross-sex marriage was the result of a strategic ethnicizing of evangelical Christian beliefs. In addition, Chinese sources demonstrate the overlapping ways that the colonial legacy in Hong Kong and Canada heavily informed Hong Kong Canadians' understandings of themselves as Hong Kong Christians in the diaspora and as racialized minorities in Canada. By analyzing interviews with key players in the debates and articles in secular and Christian Chinese publications, this chapter seeks to illuminate the discourses and decisions that produced the Hong Kong Canadian anti-same-sex marriage narrative presented to the English-speaking public.

From 2002 to 2005 Canadian political and public forums were dominated by debates about same-sex marriage. In 2002-03 three provincial courts ruled that the prohibition on same-sex marriage was an institutional violation of the Canadian Charter of Rights and Freedoms – a part of the Canadian Constitution. In response to these provincial rulings and to legal opinions from the Supreme Court of Canada that have recognized the federal government's authority to change the definition of marriage, the federal government introduced a bill in Parliament to extend federal recognition to same-sex marriages. Although this bill requires all provinces and territories to perform same-sex marriages, it prohibits religious officials from being compelled to perform such marriages. After heated debates in Parliament, the bill became law on 20 July 2005, making Canada the fourth country in the world to recognize same-sex marriages after the Netherlands in 2001, Belgium in 2004, and Spain earlier in 2005.[2] The legalization of same-sex marriage was widely regarded as accurately reflecting the opinion of the general Canadian public, with national polls showing approximately 60 percent of Canadians supporting the legislation (*Toronto Star* 2005).

In the four years leading up to the legalization of same-sex marriage, the usual players – such as conservative religious groups, lesbian and gay activists, and leaders of liberal faith traditions – came out in force to advocate for or against the proposed marriage reform. The debates also saw the emergence of new activists, among them a large contingent of Hong Kong Canadians. Hong Kong Canadians participated on all sides of the debates; many of them publicly opposed or supported the reform. At the same time, a smaller group was openly critical of the institution of marriage itself and refused to identify as either opponents or supporters of the reform. The largest group of Hong Kong Canadian activists comprised opponents of marriage reform, and they organized rallies and attended them in the thousands (see *Sing Tao* 2003a, 2004a; and *Ming Pao* 2005a). They submitted newspaper editorials to English and Chinese periodicals and held press conferences to publicize their positions to English and Chinese media outlets. As well, activists made presentations at government-organized committee meetings that sought community input on the proposed marriage bill. During this time, Hong Kong Canadians (known in English settings as "Chinese Canadians") were widely recognized as spokespeople for "ethnic" opposition to same-sex marriage in many mainstream English press and political debates.[3]

Chinese people came to Canada more than a century ago, and Hong Kong immigrants arrived in Canada en masse beginning in the 1980s. Hong Kong Canadians remain one of the largest racialized groups in the country.[4] Mobilization efforts by Hong Kong Canadians were the largest political and social campaigns orchestrated by the more than 1 million strong Chinese Canadian community. Since Hong Kong Canadians formed the largest ethnic minority in opposition to same-sex marriage in Canada and since more than half of Hong Kong Canadians in Canada – approximately 500,000 – reside in Toronto, this chapter centres on the same-sex marriage opponents in Toronto.[5] All of the Hong Kong Canadian spokespeople identified as conservative Christian, and a majority of the participants at anti-same-sex marriage gatherings belonged to evangelical Protestant churches. Most of my informants belonged to Baptist, Alliance, Free Methodist, and Chinese Community churches.[6]

Although their identity as Hong Kong Canadians was also a source of discrimination, this chapter shows that many opponents saw their nonwhite identity as a currency they could use to promote a conservative political agenda. Their ultimate goal was not just to uphold "traditional marriage" or to ensure ethnic visibility but also to re-Christianize Canada. By framing their Christian ambitions in "ethnic" terms, they were able to establish a platform to voice their religious concerns. Ultimately, they used colonial and Christian missionary discourses to articulate a new form of conservative racialized politics in Canada that was centred not on "ethnic" values but on the ethnicization of white, colonial, Christian principles.

This chapter investigates the contents and contexts of public discourses on same-sex marriage among Hong Kong Canadian opponents rather than offering a survey of general Hong Kong Canadian views on the issue. My interviews with key participants in the movement were designed strategically to find out why, how, and for whom various organizers constructed, maintained, and promoted their campaigns. Similarly, I use secular and Christian publications to highlight the public narratives that activists carefully constructed rather than to make a case about the personal conversations that took place among Hong Kong Canadians.[7]

This chapter draws from research by scholars of sexuality – including many in this volume – who view sites of sexual panics as windows through which to investigate issues that are seemingly unrelated to sex at first glance, particularly "race"-based discourses such as nationalism, colonialism, and multiculturalism. Many writers in the American and international contexts have focused on sex-based panics and controversies involving queers to produce exciting works that merge the study of nation and multiculturalism with that of sex and sexualities (Somerville 2000; see also Duggan 2003; Puar 2007; and Haritaworn 2008). Canada, I believe, provides a unique context for such an analysis.

Canada was the first Western nation to declare multiculturalism as state policy in 1971, and since then multicultural harmony has remained one of the strongest narratives that the public and government use to define Canada's nationhood.[8] Many Canadian scholars whose work is grounded in feminist and critical race theories rightfully argue that state and popular ideologies of multiculturalism have often been used to victimize Canadians of colour, particularly women and, arguably, queers (Lawrence 2004; see also Bannerji 2000; Dua 2004; and Thobani 2007).

This chapter brings discussions of religion and religious discourses to the forefront of conversations about and convergences of sex, "race," nationalism, and multiculturalism. Many Canadian "race" theorists convincingly argue that the Canadian public often stigmatizes Canadians of colour by associating them with "illiberal" religious traditions, especially non-Christian faith traditions. They are also correct to point out that many Canadians of colour use arguments of "religious and cultural authenticity" to police members in their own communities. However, a critical analysis of religious social movements organized by Canadians of colour has rarely been done. As this chapter demonstrates, a close reading of religion in the diaspora is integral when exploring nationalism, sexuality, and colonialism in Canada.

In this volume, Pamela Dickey Young, Janet Jakobsen, and Heather Shipley speak to the complicated and messy ways that religious actors declare their allegiances to the nation. Many of these actors show their patriotism by claiming their faith-based beliefs to be inherently valuable contributions to national conversations about sex and sexuality. This case study of Hong Kong Canadian Christians reveals not only that there exist multiple and frequently contradictory definitions of "nation" but also that the meaning of "allegiance" is heavily contested. What one group sees as patriotism another sees as betrayal.

This chapter first explores the narratives of divine predestination propagated by Hong Kong Canadian opponents of marriage reform. The opponents explained European colonizers' arrival in Hong Kong in the nineteenth century and Canada's multiculturalism policies in the twentieth century as parts of God's plan to prepare Hong Kongers to fight against the legalization of same-sex marriage in Canada in the early 2000s. Second, the chapter looks at the strategies used by organizers to appeal to community members' sense of Canadian nationalism. Finally, the chapter traces the legacy of European colonialism in Hong Kong and Canada in the anti-same-sex marriage narrative put forward by Hong Kong Canadian Christians. I highlight the ways that this narrative was informed heavily by the Christian vocabulary and ideology of salvation.

Discourses of Canadian Christianity and Multiculturalism

In evangelical Christian periodicals and in interviews that I conducted, many opponents saw themselves as uniquely positioned in the marriage debates and traced their position back to the history of European missionaries in China. In a call for Chinese Christians to mobilize against marriage reform, Dominic Tse (2004, 9), an evangelical Christian pastor and the most prominent spokesperson of the campaign, wrote,

> Missionaries travelled to China from the West more than a century ago because they loved the Chinese people and wished to free them from poverty, civil backwardness, and sin. They have blessed generations of Chinese by building schools and hospitals and by spreading the gospels ... In the last decades or so, God has led many Chinese people to Canada and has constructed many bible-believing and mission-minded Chinese churches.[9]

Tse claimed to speak out against homosexuality and same-sex marriage in response to God's request for "Chinese Canadian immigrants to repay our spiritual debt" through "rebuilding a morally bankrupt Canada."

Elsewhere, Tse (2003) made more explicit what he believed to be God's intention for Chinese Canadian migration by further evoking a militarist and colonizing discourse. He claimed to see Chinese Canadian churches' abundance in material and human resources as part of God's design for an "ethnic minority army in preparation for war." Tse believed that "God brought Chinese people to Canada specifically so that we can fight for his life." Through spiritual warfare, Chinese Canadian Christians would become "a new generation of nation builders" for "a divinely approved Canada."

Tse (2008) pointed to Canadian multiculturalism as forming an ideal backdrop for Chinese evangelical activism on the issues of marriage and morality. He lamented that "in the last decade or so, Canada had dismantled its Christian traditions and changed from a conservative to an extremely liberal nation on issues such as same-sex marriage, euthanasia, and abortion." Tse attributed this trend mainly to what he perceived to be the difficult positions that many white evangelicals occupy in Canada.

Tse (2008) believed that Canadian identification with multiculturalism and tolerance at the end of the twentieth century had inhibited white evangelical churches from active political engagement. As a result, many members of white evangelical churches refrained from voicing their concerns about Canadian immorality due to their fear of being labelled "homophobic" and "racist." If they were to speak up, Tse argued, the "politically correct" Canadian public would immediately dismiss them as "Anglo-Saxon Christian men" and ignore their voices.

Chinese evangelicals in Canada, however, could exploit this atmosphere. According to Tse (2008), since yellow skin had become a form of "political correctness," Chinese Christians could deliver the same moral objections as their white counterparts, and the wider Canadian populations would more willingly accept their views. Although the "local Western mainstream media may wish to challenge such positions, they would be afraid of Chinese Canadians 'playing the race card.'" In addition, since evangelical congregations make up a majority of Chinese Christians in Canada, Tse claimed that the strong organization and passion for Christian service among Chinese evangelicals made them uniquely powerful in political and social arenas. "Multiculturalism was meant to save Canada," Tse stated. "We came here because God gave Canada multiculturalism and so we have a very important mission to reshape Canada to God's liking."

However, although the fight against marriage reform was crucial, it was only part of a long-term political and spiritual campaign. The ultimate goal was to restore Canada as a Christian nation. Like Tse, many Hong Kong Canadian evangelicals regrettably noted that Canada had betrayed its Christian legacy and insisted that rampant homosexuality as well as other moral vices were signs of Canadians' demise. For instance, Richard Leung, an outreach staff in the Scarborough Chinese Baptist Church, again evoked a positive discourse of colonialism. In a letter urging the Toronto Chinese Evangelical Ministerial Fellowship (TCEMF)[10] to pursue the issue of same-sex marriage, Leung (2003) wrote: "North America, as a New World some three centuries back, was first founded by immigrants from Europe in pursuit of religious freedom and a pure Christian life. And yet when we celebrate another Canada Day, our politicians are about to dismantle the holy institution of marriage that God established for man and woman!" Similarly, columnist Lo Wai Yik (2003) lamented that "although historically North America had been the spiritual base for countless Christian missionaries, secular forces have continued to battle North American Christians."

Leung's and Lo's worry was echoed in many anti-same-sex materials circulated within Hong Kong Canadian Christian communities, and it was often coupled with an acknowledgment of the success of gay rights activism. For instance, Tse revealed that he was inspired by the effectiveness of same-sex marriage activists; recalling conversations with Chinese Canadians and Chinese pastors "brought up in Canadian systems," Tse was surprised that they used the same arguments pertaining to human rights that gay activists used.[11] In an article aimed at mobilizing Chinese Christian opposition to homosexuality, Tse (2004) asked readers to model themselves after gay activists who had "transformed successfully from a weak minority to continual victories in the span of thirty years." Tse posed the rhetorical question: "Are we ... willing to ... form God's army and reclaim Canada's spirituality in the next thirty years?"

Central to these narratives were efforts to highlight the belief that Chinese Canadian Christians' identities and experiences were distinct both from those of secular Canadians and from those of white and non-Chinese Christians in Canada. As well, many leaders' calls for collective mobilization served as a reminder that their audience's role in opposing same-sex marriage was divinely predetermined.

Many believed that God had granted them dual identities as "citizens of both heaven and earth" (Ho Cheung 2005; see also Ngai 2003; and Lo 2005). Columnist Ho Geen Wah (2003) wrote that as followers of Jesus and citizens of Canada, "we understand ... that political power originates from God and that to ... administer such power is to transport divine will to earth." Similarly, columnist Ho Cheung Oi Fai (2005) stated that "in political processes, humans are God's game tiles and humans' responsibilities are to cooperate closely with God." Like game tiles, "in every situation, we must fulfill our utmost responsibilities" and view such opportunities as "divine blessings."

Discourses of Canadian Nationalism

For many Hong Kong Canadian opponents of same-sex marriage, the driving force behind re-Christianizing Canada was their commitment to a better nation. They believed that the foundation of this commitment was laid long before Hong Kong immigrants arrived in Canada in the 1980s. For instance, Thomas Wang (2005), an American pastor who was active in the Toronto Chinese evangelical communities, highlighted the special relationship between Chinese immigrants and white Canadians in the late nineteenth century. He described Chinese labour in the construction of the Canadian railway as an example for contemporary Chinese Canadians to follow. Wang asked, "Just as Chinese workers sacrificed their lives for the Canadian railway, are Chinese Christians today willing to sacrifice themselves for building spiritual roadways connecting to other Canadians?" One way of building "spiritual roadways," according to Wang, was for Chinese Canadians to object to same-sex marriage and other forms of moral depravity. In other words, Wang asked Hong Kong Canadian Christians of the twenty-first century to see the literal nation-building efforts of earlier Chinese workers as an analogy for their current project of spiritual reconstruction.

In his call for Hong Kong Canadians to mobilize against same-sex marriage, Tse also cited examples of Chinese contributions in Canadian history. For Chinese Canadians to recognize their important roles in moral debates in contemporary Canada, Tse believed they had to learn from Chinese Canadian soldiers in the Second World War. Inspired by a visit to the graves of Chinese Canadian soldiers, he insisted that marriage campaigners, many of whom moved to Toronto in the late twentieth century, had to learn about and identify with earlier generations of Chinese Canadians. Tse claimed that in doing so they would recognize Chinese Canadians' role in building Canada and replicate this nationalistic sentiment when voicing their concerns about same-sex marriage.[12]

In addition to past nationalist endeavours, many saw Hong Kong Canadian activism in present-day Canada as especially significant and urgently needed since Chinese Canadian voices remained largely marginalized. In an editorial in a Chinese evangelical monthly distributed widely in Toronto, contributor Dat Ming (2003) recounted an unsettling experience at a rally on Parliament Hill. When he was at the event, two "Canadian elderly people" told him, "We are very excited that your Chinese contingent is part of this rally!" To Dat, these participants' seemingly gracious gesture "pointed to the institutional exclusion of Chinese Canadians and Chinese Canadians felt an urgent need for public demonstration because their voices remained unheard in the Canadian political system."

Tse shared Dat's sense of ethnic exclusion. He recalled an instance when a white, Canadian, evangelical organization had invited him to participate in a press conference in Ottawa protesting the legalization of same-sex marriage. Yet he was not given a chance to speak. Tse believed that he was asked to participate only because the evangelical group needed "a Chinese face" to "change the dynamic" between "angry white men" who lobbied against same-sex marriage and French-speaking "angry white women" journalists who supported the marriage bill. Referring to his presentation to the House of Commons on the issue of same-sex marriage in 2005 (House of Commons 2005), Tse said he believed that the Conservative Party had invited him only because it needed a token Chinese voice.[13] Elsewhere,

Tse (2005) stated that these instances of inclusion, like the idea of a multicultural Canada, were superficial and demonstrated that "Canadian multiculturalism is in big trouble." However, he insisted that the source of racialized marginalization did not lie in the *concept* of multiculturalism.

In fact, Tse stated repeatedly that the notion of multiculturalism was used unfairly against nonwhite Canadians during the marriage debates. He explained that many white Canadians saw multiculturalism as an "evil" policy that allowed immigrants to come to Canada and "water down" the white Christian tradition. He angrily pointed to such criticism as a form of white Canadian racism that accused nonwhite Canadians of contaminating Christianity and told them that they "shouldn't be here."[14]

Like Tse, TCEMF member Leung Seen Guang (2003) was also keen to defend Canadian multiculturalism. He reminded the TCEMF in a letter that it was essential that protests against same-sex marriage not be understood as opposition to multiculturalism policies. Upon hearing "shocking views in his own Christian fellowship gatherings where participants pointed to multiculturalism as a cause for same-sex marriage legalization," Leung insisted that multiculturalism was not the enemy. He noted that the policies were "the result of years of hard fought battles by minority groups who came before us." "If we attack multiculturalism," he continued, "we would be sabotaging our own campaign and alienate the rest of society." For Tse, Leung, and their allies, it was the execution, not the concept, of multiculturalism that needed to change.

To many leading opponents of same-sex marriage, however, the marriage debates were a turning point for Chinese political participation in Canadian multiculturalism. With the help of pastors like himself who acted "as prophets in the Old Testament" by giving "guidance to the flocks about major events" in their communities, Tse believed the "silent majority" of Chinese Canadians could finally speak out against same-sex marriage in an organized manner.[15] Like Tse, Dennis Mok, a pastor and one of the main organizers of anti-same-sex marriage rallies, saw that a systematic campaign provided a "proper venue" for Hong Kong Canadians to express an existing consensus about the immorality of homosexuality.[16]

According to Mok, the "proper" method of political involvement was for Hong Kong Canadians to highlight their identity as Canadians and to publicize their nationalism. During the campaign, Mok used the red and white colours "of the Canadian flag" to design t-shirts sold to Hong Kong Canadian demonstrators in order to highlight Chinese Canadian patriotism.[17] Other highly visible materials at anti-same-sex marriage demonstrations were three red banners that read, "Chinese Christian Canadians: Say NO to Defining Marriage," "Chinese Votes Count in Next Election!" and "Vote 'No' [and] You Have My Vote." As well, prior to the provincial election in October 2003 and federal elections in June 2004 and January 2006, the TCEMF and the Jubilee Centre for Christian Social Action (JCCSA), an evangelical Chinese group started by Dominic Tse in 2003,[18] held press conferences to urge Chinese Canadians to find out the positions of their political representatives on the issue of same-sex marriage (*Sing Tao* 2003c; *Ming Pao* 2004, 2006). Also, in anticipation of the three elections, the JCCSA published advertisements in all of the Chinese newspapers in Toronto with charts listing political parties' views on "moral issues," including abortion, euthanasia, pornography, and prostitution, with particular emphasis on same-sex marriage (*Sing Tao* 2003b, 2004b, 2006; *Ming Pao* 2004).

Although Tse thought that the campaigns were not as effective as he had hoped in changing the course of parliamentary discussions, he believed that after two decades of Canadian experience, Hong Kong Canadians were slowly learning "to play the game" and "speak ... in the terms that they [white Canadians] can understand." They had shown their "organizational ability, the money," and "the know-how" to influence same-sex marriage and multiculturalism policies.[19] Tse and his allies agreed that participation in marriage campaigning had transformed Toronto Hong Kong Canadians into a national force to be reckoned with.

Toward Chinese, Christian, and Canadian Authenticity

In Hong Kong Canadian Christians' anti-same-sex marriage campaign, many opponents presented cultural arguments to the English-speaking Canadian public. Within Chinese-speaking communities, however, these arguments took on an overtly religious tone. This chapter does not set out to judge which evidence or argument is "more authentic." Such a task is impossible; just as there is not and has never been a single origin or culture that is authentically "Chinese," there is no universally held set of beliefs that is authentically "Christian." Rather, the following sections of this chapter look at the multiple and nuanced ways that understandings of Chinese, Christian, and Canadian authenticities were employed to construct and further political and sexual beliefs.

Ethnicizing Christianity

Academic studies of diasporas and Canadian scholars of "race" and multiculturalism have produced a rich collection of literature addressing the homogenizing impulse of many diasporic movements in the West. Although large-scale diasporic campaigns have supported a wide spectrum of political, social, and sexual views, many narratives that have been popular among diasporic people have propagated a conservative worldview. These narratives often draw upon vocabulary that ethnicizes and essentializes cultural differences.

Works by Canadian scholars of multiculturalism Sunera Thobani and Himani Bannerji argue that diasporic appeals to authenticity and homogeneity are strategic and meant to correspond to mainstream understandings of culture, "race," and ethnic difference. Thobani (2007, 145) writes that since Canadian "multiculturalism has sought to constitute people of colour as politically identifiable by their cultural backgrounds ... race became reconfigured as culture and cultural identity became crystallized as political identity." Similarly, Bannerji (2000, 47, 45) argues that the Canadian government and public require immigrants to "speak in the state's own language of multicultural identity, of ethnicity and community" as the "only venue for social and political agency." The key way to ethnicize one's position in the multicultural setting, Bannerji (ibid., 155) explains, is to engage in "a construction of traditionality." The result, she writes, is that members of an immigrant group "engage in self-reification as ... a homogeneous whole" (ibid., 164).

Public declarations of Chinese authenticity and homogeneity, I argue, were the results of the realization by Hong Kong Canadian opponents of same-sex marriage that they must appropriate and reproduce the culturally essentialist framework of Canadian multiculturalism to secure their political, albeit marginal, inclusion in mainstream discussions. For many, the desire to be part of the English Canadian debates was made all the more urgent by everyday experiences of racial exclusion and discrimination. Both Dat Ming and Dominic Tse, for example, stated that despite the historical and current contributions by Chinese Canadians to the Christian and non-Christian communities, they were often reminded that Chinese voices were not heard or appreciated. These experiences of marginalization, I believe, further explain why effective participation in national discussions was so important to Hong Kong Canadians.

However, although the frameworks of scholars such as Bannerji and Thobani are effective in illuminating the strategies employed by Hong Kong Canadians, their analyses fall short in explaining the intentions, beliefs, and ultimate goals of these opponents of same-sex marriage. Thobani's and Bannerji's positions are premised on the argument that since people of colour participate in politics by representing their communities and positions as traditional monoliths, they only reproduce and internalize institutionalized forms of racist and colonial stereotypes. Thus they do not and cannot challenge or change a political system that is built on white supremacy. In other words, the racism embedded in the hegemonic Canadian discourses of multiculturalism would ultimately undermine or even erase the effects of their political intervention. Yet many Hong Kong Canadians referred to intentions that did not correspond neatly with those posited by Thobani, Bannerji, and other scholars of diasporic communities.

For instance, although Dominic Tse and Leung Seen Guang vigorously championed the concept of multiculturalism and although organizations like the JCCSA openly encouraged Hong Kong Canadians to participate in democratic forums, their ultimate goal was not to assimilate into Canada the way that it was but to be part of a Canada they *imagined*. This superior Canada was a Christian nation. Hence, although they recognized their democratic responsibilities, they were primarily motivated by their Christian duties to restore Canada to its former and rightful Christian glory. For Hong Kong Canadians like Mok, immoralities such as abortion, divorce, and homosexuality were evidence that Canada had lost its "Christian roots." This un-Christian and thus un-Canadian path had to be reversed. They insisted, in the words of Richard Leung (2003), that Canada must fulfil a divine destiny that began when European immigrants "founded" it "in pursuit of religious freedom and a pure Christian life."

I agree that for many Canadians of colour, the processes of essentializing "cultural" values to earn political visibility and credibility often reinforce the existing "multicultural" language of racial marginalization. Yet consideration of other frameworks shows that communities of colour do not internalize essentialist political logic in predictable ways.

Despite their public declarations of an essentialist Chinese identity, many Hong Kong Canadian opponents understood themselves, Hong Kong, and their adopted nation of Canada primarily through a Christian lens. At the same time, although they participated in the marriage debates to enhance their political influence, they saw entry into federal politics as a means to centre Christian discussions on a national stage and ultimately restore the influence of all Canadian Christians, regardless of their cultural affiliations or ethnic origins. Their understanding of Christianity was, in large part, a set of religious traditions and beliefs that stood apart from "race," even as these traditions and beliefs were propagated by racialized people like themselves.

Religious interpretations of Canadian citizenship and nationalism were most apparent in arguments for Chinese participation in elections and rallies. Columnist Ho Cheung Oi Fai (2005) reminded her readers of their dual identities as the citizens of God's community ("heaven") and Canadian society ("earth"). She was quick to point out, however, that Hong Kong Christians' democratic responsibilities were ultimately "divine blessings" that had to be used in co-ordination with God's plan. Likewise, Tse (2008) stated that Hong Kong evangelicals had to intervene in political discussions because these venues were designed to "reshape Canada to God's liking." He expressed his gratefulness to the Canadian environment of "political correctness" since it allowed Hong Kong Christians to exploit race-based anxieties. Hence his claim that "multiculturalism can save Canada" did not mean that the inclusion of Hong Kong "cultural" voices would make Canada a better place in terms of racial harmony and equality. Instead, he appealed to multicultural tolerance in the marriage debates as a way to inject Christian voices into the political arena in order to improve Canada's moral condition. Consequently, for Hong Kong Canadians like Ho Cheung and Tse, the primary differences between one political view and another, between one electoral candidate and another, and between themselves and other Canadians were not racially based. The ultimate goal of nationalistic and democratic participation was not to make Canada more Chinese per se or to stop the legalization of same-sex marriage but to rebuild Canada into a Christian nation. Conflict over same-sex marriage was simply one of the spiritual battles in a larger war.

Leading Hong Kong Canadian critics of same-sex marriage believed that God had placed Hong Kong Christians in a unique position to take charge of Canada's spirituality. In addition to their divinely blessed ability to play the "race card" (Tse 2008), many of these activists explained their God-given appointment to "save" Canada by recounting the colonial history of their place of origin. They understood British missionaries' presence in Hong Kong as paving the way for Hong Kongers to bring Christianity to Canada. For instance, Tse wrote that British missionaries had arrived in Hong Kong because "they wished to free [Chinese people] from poverty, civil backwardness, and sin"[20] and that God had destined Hong Kongers to move to Canada so that they could repay their "spiritual debt" (Tse 2004). One way to do so, according to Tse, was to protest against same-sex marriage. This narrative of British colonialism was often coupled with descriptions of British settlers bringing Christian glory to the "New World" in North America. All in all, the message of these activists was that we had to re-Christianize Canada, just as the British had made Christian converts in Hong Kong and the Europeans had saved North America through Christian conversion.

In addition to being politically positioned, many of these opponents of same-sex marriage believed that they, as immigrant Hong Kong Canadians, were uniquely endowed with authentic Christian beliefs. According to them, their "pure" and biblically accurate convictions were made especially apparent when they interacted with Canadian-born evangelicals who fell victim to Western influences and misunderstood same-sex marriage as a human right. For evangelicals like themselves, in contrast, their status as immigrants with little interaction with "liberal secular" Canada allowed them to hold on to authentic Christian beliefs and to stand firmly against homosexuality and same-sex marriage. As a result, they were able to recognize that Christians who approved of same-sex marriage were misrepresenting the Christian tradition that was once the backbone of Canada.

Intersecting Colonialisms and the Erasure of Colonial Violence

Hong Kong Canadians' imperative to missionize a spiritually inferior Canada demonstrates the complexity, adaptability, and resilience of colonial forces in a diasporic and postcolonial world. As colonized people who had travelled to a neocolonial state, Hong Kong diasporic Canadians framed their colonial experiences and the history of Canada using the language of Christian benevolence. They believed that a benevolent God had designed these destinies. As a result, they internalized and reproduced the logic and violence of British and Canadian colonizers by claiming that imperialists and their ideologies were gifts to spiritually and economically inferior worlds. To understand Hong Kong's and Canada's colonial pasts as good, many of these opponents of same-sex marriage ignored the violence and exploitation enacted during colonialism.

Britain's colonial "success" was built at the expense of the financial and political welfare of most Hong Kong residents. Beginning in the mid-twentieth century, the British and mainland governments systematically jeopardized the livelihoods of local and mainland labourers to finance Britain's and the city's industrial growth. As well, during much of British rule, Hong Kongers were denied any political representation. The highly capitalist and rather apolitical culture of Hong Kong during colonialism was, therefore, the result of the strategic exploitation of local labour and the fragmentation of political activists, not the product of the goodwill or benign presence of the colonizers (Lee 2003; see also Lau 1997; and Lo and Pang 2007).

When Hong Kong Canadians recounted the experiences of early Chinese migrants in Canada, they also downplayed the history of racial discrimination. Calling on Chinese Christians to mobilize against same-sex marriage, Wang (2005) and Tse[21] highlighted the historical relationships between Chinese immigrants and the Canadian nation-building project by citing, respectively, the examples of Chinese railway workers in the late nineteenth century and Chinese Canadian soldiers in the Second World War. This picture of Chinese Canadians willingly sacrificing for white Canadians is inaccurate and disturbing. As historical studies have shown, many Chinese workers were forcefully transported to Canada or reluctantly left China due to extreme poverty. Upon arrival, they were treated to extremely harsh working and living arrangements with little financial gain. For those who survived the railway project and decided to stay in Canada, stiff occupational restrictions confined many to demeaning jobs, and the Chinese Immigration Act (Government of Canada 1923) kept their families in China from reuniting with them in Canada (Anderson

1991; see also Li 2004, 2009). Also, works on Chinese Canadian soldiers in the Second World War have argued that many Chinese Canadians enlisted not out of appreciation for Canadian society but because they were desperate to gain state recognition as full Canadian citizens and enjoy the rights reserved only for white Canadians (Cho 2005). Hence these nation-building efforts cannot be explained simply as demonstrations of nationalistic love. They were reactions to large-scale Canadian exploitation of Chinese labour and to its legacy of racial marginalization and white supremacy.

By reimagining both the history of Chinese relations with the Canadian state and Hong Kong's colonial past, Hong Kong Canadian opponents of same-sex marriage demonstrated the pervasiveness of colonial discourses and their effectiveness in portraying colonizers as positive and benevolent. Also, these narratives showed the "success" of the colonizers in convincing the colonized that they were partners with, rather than casualties of, their invaders. More important, many opponents' convictions about the divinely ordained destinies of British colonials and Hong Kong immigrants showed the power of Christian logic to justify and reproduce colonial superiority. Although many opponents experienced racism and were aware of Canada's institutionalized ethnicization of its racialized citizens, they understood themselves as morally and spiritually superior to other non-Chinese Canadians, a conviction expressed using the colonial language of Christian missionizing. The conviction that they would eventually "triumph" through Christian faith and activism enabled many Hong Kong Canadians to make sense of their negative experiences in Canada.

Believing that God brought Hong Kongers and multiculturalism to Canada to help them carve out a "cultural" space in the marriage debates, Hong Kong Canadian Christians concluded that policies of multiculturalism, despite their ethnicizing imperative, must also be good for them. Hence, in spite of its roots in whiteness and the West, conservative Christianity's theological insistence on its moral superiority and exclusive path to salvation allowed it to be easily adapted to other racialized communities. In a twist of postcolonial fate in the Hong Kong Canadian context, the Christianizing impulse that had historically originated in the West prompted many believers to "return" to the West in order to rejuvenate their spiritual ancestors' faith. The obvious irony in the religious motivations of Hong Kong Canadian opponents of same-sex marriage was that to restore authenticity to Christianity and Canada, they had to first declare themselves to be authentically Chinese.

In addition to rewriting the histories of colonialism, many of these opponents' insistence on Canada's "Christian roots" erased the violent ways that Christianity had "arrived" and "spread." European settlers systematically eradicated Indigenous populations and cultures and exiled Indigenous communities from their land. At the same time, white settlers imposed Christianity by building churches and residential schools. Such "civilizing" endeavours have been revealed to be acts of extreme abuse and violence. Hence the repeated push for Hong Kong Christians to see early missionaries in Canada as role models for the fight against marriage reform highlighted these opponents' complicity in furthering Canada's fabricated history as a benign colonial power.

The missionary narratives were attempts to centre Chinese cultural and religious "realities," resist perceived marginalization, and claim political agency. However, in doing so, they erased the Canadian Aboriginal people, the first and ongoing victims of white Canada's colonizing efforts. Illustrating Thobani's (2007, 17) insight in her study of Canadian colonialism, Hong Kong Canadians reproduced the "complex racial hierarchy developed by colonizing powers that introduced and sustained force relations not only among settlers and Aboriginal peoples but also among the other racialized groups ranked ... as lower than whites but higher than Aboriginal peoples." Again, this demonstrated the adaptability of colonial, Christian, salvational discourses across geographic and racial lines and showed the "ease" with which colonized populations could claim these discursive forces to further marginalize other victims of colonization.

"Post"-colonial Colonialism

Closer investigation into the flexibility and power of Christian colonialist discourses in the same-sex marriage debates also sheds light on the themes of whiteness and origin central to the study of colonialism, diaspora, and religion. Many opponents re-enacted the salvational impulse of British colonizers to enhance Hong Kongers' political visibility and restore Christian and Canadian authenticity. The reproduction of colonial logic and violence is a persistent theme in scholarly works on colonial and postcolonial communities. Loomba (2005, 146), for instance, states that many currently and formerly colonized peoples read the imperialist discourse "through their own interpretive lens" when challenging colonial dominance and postcolonial conditions. Bhabha (2005, 269) argues that colonized people imperfectly mimic their colonizers just as the colonizers mimic their white counterparts back home with only partial success. Ultimately, he writes, the colonized who are "not quite/not white" inevitably become "ambivalent" subjects due to the limitations inherent in mimicry (ibid., 266, 271).

When looking at the history of Hong Kong Christians using the language of Bhabha, we can understand them as mimics of the Christian language and worldview of their British colonizers. Also, the discourse of Christianity in Hong Kong was a result of British colonial mimicry of British Christianity. Hence the Hong Kong Christian discourse became a copy of a copy of the "original" British version. In the diasporic context where Hong Kong Canadian opponents insisted on re-Christianizing Canada, their salvational arguments were necessarily imperfect copies of the Hong Kong Christian narratives since, in Bhabha's framework, transplantation necessarily produces contaminated replicas of the original. In other words, the colonial Christian discourse of Hong Kong Canadians was the copy of a copy of a copy of the "original" British version. What, then, does the study of diasporic copies of Christianity reveal about the colonizer's "original"?

Loomba (2005, 8) describes colonialism as "the conquest and control of other people's lands and goods." Colonialism is also the control of other people's epistemic access to themselves and others through the imposition of ideologies and languages. Historically, the power of colonialism rested on the primacy of white European economies, bodies, languages, and religions. Many scholars have convincingly argued that the "original" form of colonialism and, by extension, colonial Christianity functioned based on the supremacy of institutionalized whiteness (Burton 1994; see also McClintock 1995; and Stoler 2002).

Although historically Christianity's "success" in the colonies was tied to the bodies and languages of white European missionaries, large numbers of Christians in former colonies have, in turn, internalized and reproduced Christian messages of morality and salvation. This phenomenon complicates the study of the role of whiteness in contemporary Christianity. These communities' uses of the language of colonial Christianity in social and political settings are evidence that the religion's power as a colonizing tool can no longer be explained solely through its association with white superiority.

A return to Bhabha's theory of mimicry is useful to further illustrate Hong Kong Canadian Christians' relationship with white supremacy and Christianity. Although their religious discourse seemed to be a mediated copy of white, British, colonial Christianity, this diasporic copying differed from Bhabha's (2005, 267) colonized mimicry, which is "at once resemblance and menace." According to Bhabha (ibid., 266), the act of reproducing the colonial discourse by the colonized "other" creates "slippage" from the original, thus posing a threat to it. Indeed, Hong Kong Canadian opponents of same-sex marriage produced colonial narratives of Christian superiority and salvation that resembled those propagated by past colonizers. At the same time, these opponents were a menace to the "original" since the narratives challenged the authority of a foundational component of colonial Christianity, namely white colonizers as the authentic messengers of divine will. However, unlike Bhabha's subjects, who are a menace to the original by their very nature as the "other" and whose mimicry creates slippage in the very action of repetition, Hong Kong Canadian Christians' acts of rebellion were deliberate, calculated, and explicit. Hong Kong Canadian Christians openly rejected the notion that white bodies or even the proximity to whiteness necessarily conferred access to disciplinary authority and divine knowledge in the re-Christianizing agenda. Rather, they understood their otherness as central to the success of this agenda. This shows that through Christianity many opponents of same-sex marriage were able to perceive of themselves as morally superior to and thus responsible for enlightening the white "other" by means of religious conversion and education – a reproduction and inversion of the colonial worldview. Seeing white, liberal, Canadian Christians as "traitors" in the fight against same-sex marriage, many saw white Christian beliefs as inauthentic and un-Christian. In addition, using this language of Christian authenticity, many Hong Kong Canadians redrew the social hierarchy of Canada as they understood it. Rather than seeing themselves as inferior to white Canadians in a country that privileges whiteness, many felt superior to white Canadians in terms of Christian convictions. For them, being a white Canadian was often an impediment, rather than a ticket, to "true" Christianity. Thus their belief in Christianity as a set of nonracialized and universal truths helped them to understand their religious, political, and moral beliefs as not white but right.

Conclusion

During the same-sex marriage debates, Hong Kong Canadians put forth a new form of politics. Many Hong Kong Canadians intervened in the politics of multiculturalism and marriage in Canada not to ensure that their political, moral, and religious principles would be treated equally alongside those with whom they disagreed but to convince every Canadian to think exactly like them. In these marriage debates, where this new racialized form of conservative politics emerged in full force, Hong Kong Canadians used their nonwhiteness to their advantage. They erased the colonial experiences of Aboriginal Canadians and the traumatic pasts of early Chinese Canadian immigrants, all the while excusing the imperialist agendas of European missionaries in Canada and Hong Kong.

Ironically, it is precisely in the insistence on their Chineseness that whiteness is exposed as fundamental to the anti-same-sex marriage campaign of Hong Kong Canadians. Their constant return to white European Christians' colonial activities in Hong Kong and Canada was a testament to the crucial roles that white colonialism has played in constructing what it means to be a good Hong Kong Canadian Christian in present-day Canada. Understanding that the dominance and resilience of colonial power rests on white-supremacist, conservative, Christian beliefs enables us to see the intersecting legacies of colonialism in the present diasporic context. Also, recognizing that the tie between white bodies and Christianity is historically fundamental but no longer inevitable enables us to isolate the extent to which Christian beliefs and values function as colonial forces themselves.

Notes

1 Yu spoke as a representative of the Toronto Chinese Evangelical Ministerial Fellowship (TCEMF). Established by the government, the committee travelled across Canada from fall 2002 to spring 2003 in order to gather public opinion on same-sex marriage.
2 In 2004 Britain and New Zealand granted "civil partnership" and "civil union" status to same-sex couples, which are "marriage-like" laws that confer most of the rights and obligations of marriage.

3 Both Prime Minister Paul Martin and the leader of the Opposition, Stephen Harper, used Chinese Canadians as examples of communities of "ethnic Canadians" whose culture rejected same-sex marriage. Here, I use "Hong Kong Canadian" largely as a description of my subjects' places of origin or family background, and "Chinese" or "Chinese Canadian" when quoting directly from my subjects. As the chapter shows, my subjects' shifts to "Chinese Canadian" in English-language texts were highly strategic.
4 The years between the mid-1980s and the late 1990s witnessed the largest wave of Hong Kong immigration to Canada. Between 1980 and 1986 annual immigrants from Hong Kong never exceeded 10,000, but from 1986 onward the number increased dramatically, reaching 30,000 in 1990 and 44,000 in 1994. Approximately 75 percent of Hong Kong immigrants settled in Vancouver and Toronto. In the decade following 1985, emigration from Hong Kong to Canada comprised over half of all emigration from Hong Kong and approximately 16 percent of Canada's total immigration.
5 In 2006, according to census data collected by the Canadian government, 1,216,570 residents of Canada self-identified as "Chinese," and 486,330 Toronto residents self-identified as "Chinese" (Statistics Canada 2006a, 2006b).
6 I employ the language of my subjects and use the terms "Protestant" and "Christian" interchangeably. Also, whereas religious scholars differentiate between conservative and evangelical Protestant beliefs, I employ the vocabulary of my subjects and use the descriptions "evangelical" and "conservative" interchangeably.
7 In this chapter, I refer to articles published in the secular Chinese newspapers *Ming Pao Daily* (eastern Canada edition) and *Sing Tao Daily* (eastern Canada edition) and in the Christian Chinese periodicals *Association of Chinese Evangelical Ministries (ACEM) Monthly, Truth Monthly,* and *Herald Monthly*. *Ming Pao* and *Sing Tao* are the most circulated Chinese-language newspapers in Toronto, with each claiming about 100,000 readers in the city. *ACEM Monthly* is a newsletter published by Chinese Community churches across Ontario that is free to all congregants of the thirteen member churches. Depending on location, some churches, like Richmond Hill Christian Community Church, have a membership of more than 20,000. Evangelical leaders in Ontario contribute articles to this newsletter on topics ranging from Christian-centred news stories to social and political debates. *Truth Monthly* is a newspaper freely available at churches and Chinese shopping malls in the Greater Toronto Area (GTA) that reports on current Canadian social and political issues. Like *Truth Monthly, Herald Monthly* is freely available at churches and Chinese shopping malls in the GTA. Although it is an American-based publication, it is widely circulated in Canada and reports and comments extensively on Canadian issues, such as same-sex marriage.
8 In 1971 Canada declared multiculturalism to be a state policy when the Liberal government of Prime Minister Pierre Trudeau accepted all the recommendations per-

taining to multiculturalism in Volume IV of the Royal Commission on Bilingualism and Biculturalism. Trudeau stated in the House of Commons that "a policy of multiculturalism within a bilingual framework" is the "most suitable means of assuring the cultural freedom of Canadians." This policy centred on "cultural integration," and its key objectives focused on assisting "cultural groups to retain and foster their identity," "overcome barriers to their full participation in Canadian society," and "share their cultural expressions and values with other Canadians" (Dewing 2009). In 1985 the Canadian Parliament adopted the Canadian Multiculturalism Act, which remains the blueprint for major policies concerning "cultures" at the federal, provincial, and municipal levels (Government of Canada 1985). This legislation emphasizes "cross-cultural understanding and the attainment of social and economic integration through removal of discriminating barriers, institutional change, and affirmative action to equalize opportunity" (Dewing 2009).

9 My translation of the Chinese original.
10 The TCEMF began in the 1970s and is a nonprofit organization whose members are mainly Chinese Canadian and Cantonese-speaking pastors from approximately 150 evangelical Protestant churches in the Greater Toronto Area. The organization has approximately 300 members.
11 Dominic Tse, interview with author, 10 September 2008.
12 Ibid.
13 Tse, interview with author, 12 August 2008.
14 Tse, interview with author, 10 September 2008.
15 Ibid.
16 Dennis Mok, interview with author, 2 October 2008.
17 Ibid.
18 The JCCSA was established in the fall of 2003 with Tse as its executive director. Since many members of the TCEMF were refocused on their churches, Tse founded the JCCSA, and it took over the campaign. According to its website, the JCCSA has an explicitly Christian mission to "uphold social justice," "promote positive values," and "care for those who are in need on the basis of love of Christ and biblical principles." See http://www.jccsa.org.
19 Tse, interview with author, 10 September 2008.
20 My translation of the Chinese original.
21 Tse, interview with author, 10 September 2008.

References

Anderson, K.J. 1991. *Vancouver's Chinatown: Racial Discourse in Canada, 1875-1980*. Montreal and Kingston: McGill-Queen's University Press.

Bannerji, H. 2000. *The Dark Side of the Nation: Essay on Multiculturalism, Nationalism and Gender*. Toronto: Canadian Scholars' Press.

Bhabha, H.K. 2005. Of Mimicry and Man: The Ambivalence of Colonial Discourse. In *Postcolonialisms: An Anthology of Cultural Theory and Criticism*, ed. G. Desai and S. Nair, 265-73. New York: Rutgers.

Burton, A. 1994. *Burdens of History: British Feminists, Indian Women, and Imperial Culture, 1865-1915*. Chapel Hill: University of North Carolina Press.

Cho, Karen. 2005. *In the Shadow of Gold Mountain*. Documentary. National Film Board of Canada.

Dat, Ming. 2003. Beginning with the Provincial Election. *Toronto Herald Monthly*, October, 14.

Dewing, M. 2009. Canadian Multiculturalism. 15 September. http://www.parl.gc.ca/Content/LOP/ResearchPublications/2009-20-e.htm.

Dua, E. 2004. Racializing Imperial Canada: Indian Women and the Making of Ethnic Communities. In *Sisters and Strangers? Immigrant, Ethnic, and Racialized Women in Canadian History*, ed. M. Epp, F. Iacovetta, and F. Swyripa, 71-88. Toronto: University of Toronto Press.

Duggan, L. 2003. *The Twilight of Equality? Neoliberalism, Cultural Politics, and the Attack on Democracy*. Boston: Beacon.

Government of Canada. 1923. *Chinese Immigration Act*.

–. 1985. *Canadian Multiculturalism Act*, c. 24 (4th Supp.).

Haritaworn, J. 2008. Loyal Repetitions of the Nation: Gay Assimilation and the "War on Terror." *darkmatter*, 2 May. http://www.darkmatter101.org/site/2008/05/02/loyal-repetitions-of-the-nation-gay-assimilation-and-the-war-on-terror.

Ho, G.W. 2003. "Becoming Flesh" – Role Model for Christian Social Engagement. *ACEM Monthly*, November, 5.

Ho Cheung, O.F. 2005. Christians and Politics. *Truth Monthly*, February. http://www.truth-monthly.com/issue137/0502pf04.htm.

House of Commons. 2005. *Edited Hansard* (058), 38th Parliament, 1st Session (16 February): 1520-1740.

Lau, S.-K. 1997. *Decolonization without Independence and the Poverty of Political Leaders in Hong Kong*. Hong Kong: Hong Kong Institute of Asia-Pacific Studies.

Lawrence, B. 2004. *"Real" Indians and Others: Mixed-Blood Urban Native Peoples and Indigenous Nationhood*. Vancouver: UBC Press.

Lee, E.W.Y., ed. 2003. *Gender and Change in Hong Kong: Globalization, Postcolonialism, and Chinese Patriarchy*. Vancouver: UBC Press.

Leung, S.G. 2003. TCEMF, Mok Papers. Documents in the author's possession.

Li, P.S. 2004. Chinese. In *The Oxford Companion to Canadian History*, ed. G. Hallowell. http://www.oxfordreference.com.

–. 2009. Chinese. In *The Encyclopedia of Canada's Peoples*, ed. Multicultural History Society of Ontario. http://www.multiculturalcanada.ca/Encyclopedia/A-Z/c10.

Lo, K.-C., and L. Pang. 2007. Hong Kong: Ten Years after Colonialism. *Postcolonial Studies* 10 (4): 349-56.

Lo, W. 2005. Protect Our Noble Tradition, Steer Next Generations to the Right Path. *Truth Monthly,* August. http://www.truth-monthly.com/issue143/0508sn03.htm.

Lo, W.Y. 2003. "Must Not Ignore the Current Crisis." *Truth Monthly,* August. http://www.truth-monthly.com/issue119/0308mt02.htm.

Loomba, A. 2005. *Colonialism/Postcolonialism.* 2nd ed. London: Routledge.

McClintock, A. 1995. *Imperial Leather: Race, Gender, and Sexuality in the Colonial Contest.* New York: Routledge.

Ming Pao. 2004. Protect Traditional Marriage: Chinese Religious Group Urges Chinese to Vote Carefully. 22 June, A3.

–. 2005a. Coalition Advocates Name Change to "Marriage." 13 July, A3.

–. 2005b. Only Chinese Participant at Same-Sex Marriage Hearing. 21 May, A1.

–. 2006. JCCSA Urges Chinese Christians to Vote on Moral Values. 12 January, A3.

Ngai Lau, K. 2003. Urgent! Please Act Now! *Truth Monthly,* August. http://www.truth-monthly.com/issue119/0308mt03.htm.

Puar, J.K. 2007. *Terrorist Assemblages: Homonationalism in Queer Times.* Durham, NC: Duke University Press.

Sing Tao. 2003a. Close to 10,000 Chinese Christians Gather at Queen's Park to Protest Same-Sex Marriage Legislation. 7 September, A9.

–. 2003b. Firmly Protect One-Man-One-Woman Marriage. 27 September, A19.

–. 2003c. TCEMF Continues to Collect Anti-Same-Sex Marriage Letters, Urges Chinese to Voice Concerns in Federal Election. 19 September, A7.

–. 2004a. Chinese Religious Organization Supports One-Man-One-Woman Marriage. 6 October, A4.

–. 2004b. Support One-Man-One-Woman Marriage, Vote for Politicians Who Share Your View. 22 June, A15.

–. 2006. Federal Election, 123! Vote! Protect your Traditional Values. 15 January.

Somerville, S.B. 2000. *Queering the Color Line: Race and the Invention of Homosexuality in American Culture.* Durham, NC: Duke University Press.

Statistics Canada. 2006a. Visible Minority Groups, 2006 Counts, for Canada and Census Metropolitan Areas and Census Agglomerations – 20% Sample Data. http://www12.statcan.ca/census-recensement/2006/dp-pd/hlt/97-562/pages/page.cfm?Lang=E&Geo=CMA&Code=01&Table=1&Data=Count&StartRec=1&Sort=2&Display=Page.

–. 2006b. Visible Minority Groups, 2006 Counts, for Canada, Provinces and Territories – 20% Sample Data. http://www12.statcan.ca/census-recensement/2006/dp-pd/hlt/97-562/pages/page.cfm?Lang=E&Geo=PR&Code=01&Table=1&Data=Count&StartRec=1&Sort=2&Display=Page.

Stoler, A.L. 2002. *Carnal Knowledge and Imperial Power: Race and the Intimate in Colonial Rule.* Berkeley: University of California Press.

Thobani, S. 2007. *Exalted Subjects: Studies in the Making of Race and Nation in Canada.* Toronto: University of Toronto Press.

Toronto Star. 2005. Canadians Split over Same-Sex Marriage. 12 February, A1, A4.

Tse, D. 2003. Arise, a New Generation of Nation Builders! *ACEM Monthly*, November, 1-3.

–. 2004. "At All Cost!" – Religious Reflection on Bill C-250. *ACEM Monthly*, April, 9.

–. 2005. Not Admitting Defeat – Reflections on the Passing of Same-Sex Marriage Bill. *ACEM Monthly*, September, 3.

–. 2008. Multiculturalism Can Save Canada! Interview with Pastor Dominic Tse from Canada's Jubilee Centre for Christian Social Action. *Christian Times*, 31 August.

Wang, T. 2005. No More Silence. *Truth Monthly*, April. http://www.truth-monthly.com/issue139/0504mt02.htm.

PART 2

**Sexuality and the Construction
of Religious Identities**

SEXUALITY HAS A significant effect on the construction of religious identities, as the chapters in this section demonstrate. There is no one static and essential meaning of religion or religious identity, yet there is a North American societal tendency to conflate religion with a conservative, evangelical Christianity that is heteronormative. Further, as will become evident throughout this section, the point of connection between sexual identity and religious identity has become a common location of moral panic.

The effects of sexuality discourse on religious identities and identity formation cannot be adequately discussed without also considering the reverse: the effects of religious discourse on sexual identities and identity formation. Further, neither can be adequately considered without attention to contextual factors, including systemic power distribution as well as political and other interest groups. For example, socio-political religious conflicts stir up intense emotions and tend to devolve into rights-based arguments that privilege the systemically more powerful and that often ignore or compromise the agency of marginalized individuals and groups.

The authors in this section are clear that a sacred-profane bifurcation is a false construction; religious identity formation is dynamic, ongoing, and connected to both society and the individual. Religious identity is affected by socio-political norms and by personal sexual experiences that can conflict with these norms. In the chapters in this section, Heather Shipley, Andrew Kam-Tuck Yip, and Catherine Holtmann all highlight the ambiguity of religion as an influential factor in sexual identity formation. As will become clear throughout this section, these challenges can lead to wider socio-political reconstructions.

This section provides a rich sampling of methodological approaches to identity formation, including sociological quantitative and qualitative analysis, narrative illustrations, postmodern theory, queer theory, and spatial theory. This collection of three chapters provides a rich teaching tool with which to introduce readers to the ramifications of sexuality and religion for micro and macro identity formation. Imagination and resilience emerge as resources for reshaping a more diverse and inclusive world.

In Chapter 4, Heather Shipley explores identity struggles in her analysis of the proposal for, and reactions against, changes to the teaching of sexuality in the Ontario provincial education curriculum. In particular, she addresses the ways that identity is "regulated, managed, and constructed" through public policy and media discourse.

Shipley arrives at the insight that the oppositional construction of essentialized religious and sexual identities is one of the most significant causal dynamics of the sex education issue. Similar to both Yip and Holtmann (and in the first section, Pamela Dickey Young), she examines the tendency to reduce what is meant by religious identity to a one-dimensional typology that is opposed to any sexually progressive education and resistant to sexual diversity.

Shipley turns to a creative consideration of spatial theory and posits that if school space belongs in large part to the youth and children who are students, their voices (agency) and identities ought to factor into the debate over the sex education curriculum. Public controversy over hot-button topics (locations of moral panic) often devolves into rights-based arguments exclusive of value and contextual analysis, as we see illuminated throughout this anthology. The question of whose agency is accorded most or least power is very political and is strongly related to issues of identity, as Shipley demonstrates in this loaded and timely case.

In Chapter 5, Andrew Kam-Tuck Yip looks at the intersection between sexuality and religion in the context of the diktat of sex only within marriage. Methodologically, he draws on both qualitative and quantitative research, with constructive themes emerging from his in-depth studies of lesbian, gay, and bisexual (LGB) Christians, Muslims, and Buddhists, as well as heterosexual and LGB religious young adults of diverse religious faiths. Reinforcing Shipley's contention, Yip acknowledges the widespread construction and perception of religion as antithetical to sexual diversity. This chapter's attention is on subjects' diverse experiences in managing these identity tensions and on their social and political implications. As does Holtmann, Yip contests the bifurcation between the sacred and the profane, the spirit and the body, pointing to the narratives of many subjects who insist on the interconnection of their sexual and religious identities; it is this connection that results in angst and often shame, evoking conflict when these components of one's identity are at odds.

Yip's research, similar to Shipley's, points to the role of normative religious sexual codes, including the conservative Christian norm of sex only within heterosexual marriage, in creating identity conflicts. Like Holtmann, Yip discovered that subjects use diverse coping strategies in response to identity conflict and tension. Particularly among LGB subjects who desire to be part of a religious group but are not fully accepted because of their sexual identities, commonly employed coping strategies include the compartmentalization of one's sex and faith lives, leaving one's religion, suppressing one's sexuality, and abstaining from sex.

Yip concludes with the insight that identity tensions can lead to religious, social, and political transformation when these actors claim their own positive experiences, reject shaming messages, and take pride in who they are, knowing that the divine accepts and loves them. The identities of LGB religious actors can challenge constructions of religion and society as well as of the Divine.

In Chapter 6, Catherine Holtmann considers the Roman Catholic Church's responses to domestic violence and the implications of these responses for women's reproductive choices, focusing on the Roman Catholic Church in Canada. Holtmann's review of Catholic social policy exposes contradictions particularly between the papal commitment to "right to life" and an apparent lack of commitment to women's lives and embodied well-being. Holtmann argues that the right to life of the unborn fetus appears to take priority over the right to life of the mother in the Roman Catholic Church, as does the sanctity of heterosexual marriage over women's right not to be abused. Holtmann points out that although divorce is recognized by Rome as legitimate in cases of abuse and violence, priests seem to do little to educate and preach on the sin of this violence. She draws a complex picture of Catholic social policy, observing that although generally the exercise of women's agency within the Roman Catholic Church is systemically difficult, there are some exceptions, particularly within the Canadian context.

These paradoxical and devaluing messages have created tensions in the lives of Roman Catholic women. Holtmann explores these tensions through an analysis of narratives collected from over 100 Canadian Catholics. These tensions and conflicts, similar to those outlined in both Shipley's and Yip's chapters, create identity struggles for women who self-identify as Roman Catholic and who experience their embodied and sexual identities as incongruent with and marginalized by many of the dictates that inform their religious identity. Problematizing these tensions are experiences of domestic violence.

Through the study of collected narratives, Holtmann concludes that there are four main strategies women use to reimagine and construct their religious and sexual identities and to reclaim their agency: "(1) placing people before principles, (2) resisting a culture of silence, (3) fostering ministries of caring, and (4) building movements of religious change."

– Tracy J. Trothen

4

Challenging Identity Constructs
THE DEBATE OVER THE SEX EDUCATION CURRICULUM IN ONTARIO

Heather Shipley

This chapter takes its inspiration from the changes to the Ontario sex education curriculum proposed in 2010, changes that elicited a fair amount of controversy in the media and that were subsequently put on hold for further review. This chapter examines the current curriculum, the proposed changes, the controversy following the proposal, and the challenges posed when the topics of sex, sexuality, and sex education make their way into public discourse. At the heart of much of my work is the desire to find ways to bridge gaps between important and cutting-edge theoretical work regarding identity and identity constructions and the ways that identity is regulated, managed, and constructed within systems of authority, such as schools, policy, legislation, and so on. Here, I bring together theoretical work from an interdisciplinary perspective regarding religion, sexuality, and ideologies and use the debate over the sex education curriculum in Ontario to illustrate how little of the theoretical work on the complexity of identity constructs makes its way into debates and controversies in media and public discourse. I am interested in thinking through how we connect identities, such as religious and sexual identities, so that they are seen as less essentialized and less oppositional in media and public discourses.[1]

My argument follows on the theme of this collection by pushing the boundaries of both the religious and the sexual to discuss the ways that some religious groups and individuals frame opposition to teaching about sexuality and about certain kinds of sexuality,[2] how all religious groups are subsequently purported to be unified under the same ideologies, and how sexual diversity and sexuality still elicit so much response that simple adjustments to education curricula can be revised, regardless of content, consultation, or requirement. This discussion builds on other controversies over gay and lesbian teachers, which are illustrated by the Little Flower controversy in British Columbia (*CBC News* 2010a),³ and thematically follows the analysis of the modifications to the Alberta Human Rights Act introduced in Bill 44 (Government of Alberta 2009), which Pamela Dickey Young examines in detail in Chapter 2 of this volume.

I reflect on the following questions in response to the controversy over the Ontario sex education curriculum. How do individuals learn and/or teach about sex, gender, and sexuality? When an educator or parent is teaching about sex, gender, and sexuality, what are they at the same time teaching about religion, religious ideology, and religious identity, and correspondingly what is the student learning? And, in light of controversies such as the sex education curriculum, Little Flower, and Bill 44, what are individuals willing to teach, and what do they expect students to learn?

Theory and Identity

In this chapter, I briefly outline the spatial dimensions of the curriculum debate, an important element requiring further analysis, and specifically ask whose voices are given power and whose are silenced. Kim Knott's (2009) analysis of the spatial dimensions of any experience includes (1) how it is perceived, (2) how it is conceived, and (3) how it is lived. I am interested in the perception of the space of education when examining these debates and in what dominant norms and voices influence the shape of identity assumptions and impositions. I will reflect on the voices that are given space within this debate and question those that remain silent.

Knott uses work of geographers such as Henri Lefebvre and David Harvey, both of whom incorporate analysis of the power relations and dynamics encompassed in space and place, to discuss the spatial location of religion as a means of analyzing data. Knott (2009, 162) states: "Spatial methodology entails a consideration of the dynamism of the object or place, first by means of its spatial *aspects* – the way in which it is practiced, represented and lived ... – and, secondly, by means of the processes of production and reproduction that form it and allow it to generate new spaces" (emphasis in original).

In this particular case, the site of school is conceived not only at a policy level (education policy and education curriculum) but also at a physical, geographical level (the building in which policies are enacted, teachers work, and students are socialized and educated). It is lived by a number of participants, including the principals, teachers, students, and parents of students in various ways. The lived experience of the space of school is a dynamic process of interaction between individuals and groups who are involved in the space, whether daily or only occasionally. For the purposes of this chapter, my interest is primarily in how the space becomes "owned" by dominant voices in the media and how the perception of this space is then transferred from students, teachers, administrators, and policy makers to those who are most vocal in public discourse on the subject.

It is evident in reading through media coverage of these debates that the sex education curriculum is perceived by many individuals and groups as part of their lived experience even though they are not teachers or students and in some cases are not parents of students either. Although some parents' voices certainly were involved in the discussions, much of the controversy covered in the media in April 2010 involved groups and individuals who were not necessarily parents of students, or teachers, or administrators, or principals, or policy makers. Although Ontario premier Dalton McGuinty declared that the curriculum changes must be put on hold to consider the diversity of the province, it is clear that only some voices were heard and given power, those of organizations such as Canada Christian College and the Institute for Canadian Values, not a spread of diverse voices. Others' voices were either ignored or not heard at all. The space of the debate was removed from the education institution, and ownership of the space of the education curriculum ended up resting with a small group.

Norms and identity impositions are evidenced through (1) critique of law as a narrative script (e.g., Amsterdam and Bruner 2000), (2) the formulation of public policy (e.g., Dickey Young, Chapter 2, this volume; Jakobsen and Pellegrini 2008), and (3) the management and regulation of identity norms in education, a focus of this chapter. It has been repeatedly demonstrated in social sciences and humanities and increasingly in scientific study that identity negotiation and understanding are complex and diverse and consistently shift over a lifetime (e.g., Foucault 1978, 1985,

1988; Butler 1993; Burn 1996; Kinsey 1998a, 1998b; Gleason 1999; Suh 2002; Dickey Young 2008; Yip, Chapter 5, this volume).

Queer theory is an approach to identity that can be used to address the challenges posed by the essentialization of identity in media and public discourses. Embracing the term "queer," which is often applied derogatorily to gay and lesbian individuals, queer theorists examine the production of normal and dominant approaches in the organization of sexuality as a category of identity, most often in the management of sexuality. Although there is not one singular approach or disciplinary venue from which queer theory stems, the project of queer theory examines sexuality not as an intrinsic or inherent trait but by critiquing "discursive productions of sexual identity" (Schippert 2005, 91) in relation to other categories of meaning. As others point out (e.g., Duggan and Hunter 2006), queer theory itself can be seen as a normalized discourse, reframing the categories of difference within a heterosexual vernacular. Denike (2010) critiques what she argues is the creation of "homonationalist" identities, subsequently used to create new "others." However, the necessity of a project of queering stereotypes and assumptions is demonstrated by examining education policies, such as the sex education curriculum. Certain categories of identity (gender identity and sexual orientation) are framed as problematic inclusions in the curriculum because of their association with non-normative identities and orientations.

Sexual and religious identities can quickly become reduced by an essentialist approach, through which individuals become identified solely as the category into which their religious or sexual identification fits. Identity essentialism is often framed within a rigid standpoint, legally and socially, that does not allow for possibilities across set boundaries of identity. This essentialism permits for an approach in which humans are framed solely as these set categories of identity, which "narrow our field of vision ... [because we do not] experience this complex world as only a gender or a race or a class or a nationality or a sexuality, and so on" (Winnubst 2006, 17).

Despite assumptions that have often been made about static sexual identities, studies have shown that individuals live their religious and sexual identities through a constant negotiation among aspects of identity, social norms, and shifting cultural experiences (e.g., Wilcox 2010; Yip, Chapter 5, this volume). Such varied theoretical analyses regarding identity often do not make their way into the public arena when debates about sex, sexuality, and religion are at the forefront of public controversy.[4] As a result, identity challenges and debates become posited as a "clash" between the right to freedom of religion and equality rights based on sex, gender, and sexual orientation, all posited as given and unchanging. This essentialism leaves no room for the possibility that individuals can be religious and in support of teaching about healthy sexuality in the classroom (among other possibilities regarding sexuality). Rather, "the" religious voice is framed as being opposed to or under threat by sex, gender, and sexuality. The space of these debates, whether in media or public discourse, produces specific rigid identity formations regarding what it means to "be" religious – and correspondingly places discussions about sex and sexuality in contrast to "being" religious.

There is a wide body of literature on the discrepancies between religious texts and lived religion, or between what religion is assumed to be and how people practise their faith by contextualizing doctrine based on their own needs, experiences, and cultural influences (e.g., McGuire 2008; Wilcox 2010).[5] These discrepancies demonstrate one part of the puzzle to be considered in examining the fluidity of religious ideologies across and within religious groups. As diverse religious groups continue to cohabit in closer proximity to one another, it becomes increasingly evident in public discourse that there is no one unified understanding of what being religious means. This fact can be demonstrated by analyzing the diverse ways that people engage with their religious beliefs, whether by going to a church or a mosque, through home worship, or by living according to a system of ethics (see Beyer 2008).

Incorporating the theoretical analyses outlined above to examine identity fluidity, I think about education and, in particular, curriculum both as spaces conceived by systems of authority (further evidenced by political decisions regarding curriculum) and as lived and perceived spaces of students and youth. The school, although imposed on children, is also their space – of interaction, education, and socialization – and provides a fundamental space for identity formation. The implications of the conceived, perceived, and lived aspects of space (see Knott 2009), included here as part of this discussion of the sex education curriculum, inform the complexity of this discussion – and also highlight what appears to be a complete negation of an active role for students in a discussion of their education curriculum. We have heard from politicians, academics, special-interest groups, and parents; space also needs to be made in the debate to determine how students feel about the sex education component of their education.[6]

Proposed Changes

In the spring of 2010, Ontario premier Dalton McGuinty[7] was faced with questions about proposed changes to the Ontario sex education curriculum that some believe he was not anticipating (*CBC News* 2010b). McGuinty's first response was to defend the curriculum, saying that children as young as eight years of age should be learning about various issues, including gender identity and sexual orientation. In the aftermath of his defence, however, the premier backed off the curriculum changes, which have since been postponed and are under review. Notably, the timeline of events is incredibly brief: McGuinty was first asked about the changes on 21 April; he had reversed his opinion regarding the proposed changes by 23 April.

Some of the revisions to the curriculum, which had been slated for implementation in the fall of 2010, were as follows: Grade 1 students were to be taught to identify genitalia using the correct words, such as "penis," "vagina," and "testicle";[8] Grade 3 students would learn about gender identity and sexual orientation, the first time these subjects were specified in the Ontario curriculum, along with other invisible differences (such as allergies); Grade 5 students were to be taught to identify parts of the reproductive system and describe how the body changes during puberty; Grade 6 students were to learn about masturbation and wet dreams; and Grade 7 students would be taught about oral and anal sex and about how to prevent unintended pregnancy and sexually transmitted infections, including HIV. These changes had been suggested as necessary to adapt to contemporary standards of sexual health education and to increase understanding regarding sexual identity; the new topics were intended to be introduced to students at age-appropriate and developmentally relevant stages in their education.

Depending on the media outlet one is accessing, the language of "who" is being taught changes: from students to children and kids. The intention is fairly obvious; using terms such as "children" and "kids" implies individuals far too young to be discussing penises, vaginas, oral sex, or sexual orientation. Describing students as "kids" or "children" also implies a moral component, further emphasizing the assumption of the vulnerability of those to whom this curriculum would apply. Reactions to these changes often did not take into account the actual proposed changes. Thus some responses spoke as though Grade 1 students were to be taught about anal sex. No level of insistence that Grade 1 students would in fact learn only the appropriate names for body parts – which they actually possess, one presumes – could appease some of the opponents of changes to the sex education curriculum or quell their outrage at what "their" children would be exposed to.[9]

Alex McKay of the Sex Information and Education Council of Canada noted,

> It is developmentally appropriate for students in Grade 3 to have an awareness that not all people are heterosexual ... Before any type of education takes place in the schools, many kids are going to be walking through the doors with that awareness anyway. The curriculum is appropriate and knowledge is preferable to ignorance ... The issue is that we live in a culture that is saturated with sexual imagery and that it is more important than ever that young people have a solid foundation of basic knowledge about human development and sexuality, and that this curriculum helps to deliver that. It would be compromising the health and well-being of our youth if we shy away from providing this important information and skill set. (Nguyen 2010)

The current health curriculum in Ontario states:

> Parents and guardians are the primary educators of their children. As children grow and develop relationships with family members and others, they learn about appropriate behaviours and values, as well as about sexuality. They are influenced by parents, friends, relatives, religious leaders, teachers, and neighbours, as well as by television, radio, videos, movies, books, advertisements, music, and newspapers. School-based programs add another important dimension to a child's ongoing learning about sexuality. (Ontario Ministry of Education 1998, 10)

The Ontario curriculum already outlines the need to respect individual differences and to make parents and guardians aware of the content of the curriculum and timing of delivery. What would have been different if the proposed changes had taken effect was the specification of the topics to be addressed within the different grades; the curriculum right now is vague, which has allowed for broad interpretation (see ibid.). McKay argued that the proposed changes would have brought the Ontario curriculum in line with other curricula in Canada (Nguyen 2010). Although this claim is not entirely accurate, with different provinces approaching the topic of sex education in various ways, the process of developing these changes for Ontario was carefully done and included consultation with health and education experts and parents, to be discussed in more detail below.

In the existing curriculum and guide regarding the "Growth and Development" portion of the health curriculum, human reproductive processes are first mentioned in Grade 3; characteristics of healthy relationships in Grade 4; puberty changes in Grade 5, as well as menstruation and spermatogenesis; the relation of changes at puberty to reproductive organs and dealing with peer pressure in Grade 6; male and female reproductive systems and fertilization, STDs, and abstinence as it applies to healthy sexuality in Grade 7; and the importance of abstinence as a positive choice, symptoms and methods of transmissions of STDs, pregnancy prevention, and living skills related to sexual activities (and the use of drugs) in Grade 8. In the later years, it is also emphasized that students should be able to identify sources of support regarding healthy sexuality such as parents, guardians, and doctors. Clearly, the differences in the proposed curriculum are the specific mentions of body parts and sexual acts as well as the inclusion of discussing sexual and gender identity.

The process by which these changes were formulated began in 2007 and included a year of research and consultation with public and Catholic school boards, university faculties of education, health groups, and parent groups. The first draft of the proposal was sent out for public feedback, resulting in 3,000 responses that subsequently led to further revision and fact-checking prior to finalizing the proposed changes in 2009 (Benzie 2010). Annie Kidder of the parent group People for Education also noted that the new curriculum had been circulated to 5,000 parents in Ontario, many of whom she said were supportive of the changes as indicating adaptation to the twenty-first century (Howlett and Hammer 2010).

Responses: The Institute for Canadian Values and Canada Christian College
Public responses to the proposed changes were rapid after they were announced in 2010. Reverend Ekron Malcolm, with the Institute for Canadian

Values, stated that he and other "family-focused" groups had launched a campaign against the curriculum and were organizing a protest in Toronto for 10 May 2010. Malcolm and Charles McVety, president of Canada Christian College, started an online petition against the proposed changes. Malcolm stated: "I can't imagine a child now has to question their gender, question their identity ... I think there's enough confusion among our children in the world, for them now having to question themselves. This is where I would draw the line" (Nguyen 2010). Malcolm argued against the topic of sexual diversity in elementary schools and also objected to teaching about oral and anal sex: "Schools don't need to be teaching my children about sexual orientation or sex education. Those decisions should be left to the family, to the parents, to guide children. These topics can be taught at the high school level, at the university level, when children can make up their minds" (ibid.).

Murielle Boudreau, of the Greater Toronto Catholic Parent Network, also opposed the proposed changes and was part of a consolidated effort by some Christian and Muslim groups threatening to pull their children out of school in order to protest the changes. Boudreau stated that the new information would "traumatize these children – they're going to be doing everything out in the school yard" (*Maclean's* 2010).

I am aware that sensational debates and voices help to "sell" the news, so the same oppositional voices are regularly polled regarding specific debates. However, it is important to consider the possibility that other voices would be valid in these controversies. Media coverage of "the religious" response to the sex education curriculum focused exclusively on religious individuals or groups that opposed the curriculum,[10] demonstrating again the problematic privileging of "the religious" voices that are presented as universally representative in Canada, without consideration of groups or individuals who are both religiously identified and also support teaching about healthy sexuality, gender identity, or sexual orientation in the classroom. Importantly, Nason-Clark (Chapter 9, this volume) raises questions about the location of moral panics within a society. She points out that often the moral panics represented in public and media discourses reflect particular viewpoints at particular times and tend to reaffirm one ideological set of values. Through the assumption of identity essentialism, much of the April 2010 media coverage of the sex education curriculum placed gender identity and sexual orientation at the forefront of Canada's radar of moral panic, although Ontarians in general might well have held a much broader view overall.[11]

The media's continued positioning of "the religious" as standing in opposition to sexuality – in this case, in the form of sex education – demonstrates a particular moral panic concerning sex, sexuality, and sexual diversity within a Canadian context. This assumption about the standing of religion reaffirms not only that it is acceptable for "the religious" to oppose the teaching of sexuality but also that religious groups and individuals are expected to feel this way. This view, in turn, fuels a larger societal moral panic about religion, sex, and sexuality – topics that are individualized and personalized in a way that math or science are not.

During the debate, an article in the *National Post* included an interview with Elizabeth Schroeder, executive director of Answer, an organization at Rutgers University that promotes comprehensive sexuality education. Schroeder said that when she saw McGuinty change his mind regarding the curriculum changes, she "thought: Oh great, why don't you just move down here. That's what we do in the States, kow-tow to parents groups and religious leaders instead of sticking our feet in the ground and saying 'We are the educational experts'" (McParland 2010). Dickey Young's analysis of Bill 44 in Chapter 2 of this volume ties into the discussion of moral panics and the expectations of "the religious." Identity is not seen as the purview of select fields of expertise the way that science and math are, so teaching about religion and sexuality takes on a further complexity, evidenced in the debates about the sex education curriculum and about modifications to the Alberta Human Rights Act introduced in Bill 44 (Government of Alberta 2009). Public consultation is not sought when changes are made to areas of teaching that are not identity-based, and therefore perhaps less controversial, because the expectation is not that everyone is an expert regarding other topics taught in school. But, as Dickey Young posits, perhaps the link that is drawn between these categories, which continually places them together in these controversial debates, is the link to identity: we are all "experts" regarding religious and sexual identity by the fact of our individual understanding of our own religion or sexuality.

I have included Malcolm's, McVety's, and Boudreau's responses here because they are the voices represented most often in the media to indicate a certain notion of "moral opposition" regarding sexuality and sexual diversity. The privileging of these voices illustrates a problematic at the heart of this work; how and when do we make room for other religious voices in debates within Canadian media and public discourses – how do we connect other religious identities? In other public controversies, such as the same-sex marriage reference in 2005, it was clear in the list of interveners that a number of religious organizations and individuals supported the right to marriage for same-sex couples. And as evidenced by religious organizations such as the United Church of Canada and Salaam Canada,[12] not all religious groups are unified in their opposition to sexuality and sexual diversity.[13]

Yet, in the media and in public decision making, the space of this education debate shifted toward voices of groups, such as the Institute for Canadian Values, Canada Christian College, and the Greater Toronto Catholic Parent Network, rather than focusing on students, on the teachers who would be implementing the new policy in the classroom, or on groups, including religious groups, that might favour the new curriculum. Certain voices became dominant in a debate about a curriculum that is spatially not centred on them.

What Do the Parents Say?

Responses from parents to the proposed changes to the sex education curriculum were diverse, with some strongly opposed and others arguing that the changes would provide necessary and important education regarding sexuality. On 23 April 2010 *CBC News* (2010c) quoted three different parental responses to the debate over the sex education curriculum. Rehana Shaik stated, "I don't want the kids at a tender age to learn all that sex education. My younger son will be starting Grade 1 next year and I don't want him to learn all that." Rosalinde Rundle said that she wanted her child to be comfortable with sexuality, arguing, "They'll learn [sex education] in school, and then every kid will learn the same thing, and then they won't make such a big deal of it probably, because it's not so taboo." And Sherri-Anne Medema was critical of McGuinty's change of heart, stating, "It goes beyond religious beliefs. It goes beyond what culture the people are from, and [McGuinty] should stick to his guns and say, 'OK, we're going to continue on.'"

For some, the question of sex education remained framed as a cultural problem. As Medema noted, although groups from certain "cultures" (presumably not "Canadian" culture) were likely to be opposed, there should not be any accommodation or modification in response.[14] The prominent religious voices that were quoted as opposing the changes to the curriculum – Canada Christian College and the Institute for Canadian Values – are not representative of religious or cultural minorities in Canada. Contemporary debates about religion and culture, and religious accommodation, which are highly contested subjects in other arenas in Canada, became interwoven in a discussion about sex education. And although some sources (see Rayside 2010) suggested that "Muslim groups" were also opposed to the changes, the Muslim association repeatedly named in the lists of opponents was the Somali Parents for Education. Rayside (ibid.) has examined the influence of religious mobilizing on policy, with a particular eye to the sex education curriculum in Ontario. He analyzes the role of multiple religious organizations but states that there was also a "push back from among 'new Canadians' – communities with large numbers of immigrants who had traditionally voted Liberal" (ibid., 13). Although this "push back" is not evident in the media coverage per se, with the quotations coming in large part from McVety and Malcolm and from the websites and protests organized by them and their organizations, the public perception somehow began to be that the curriculum was halted by "new Canadians." It didn't matter, as illustrated in the coverage outlined in this chapter, that the rest of the groups who expressed their concerns were all Christian-based organizations, not minority-group associations (Hammer and Howlett 2010a; McParland 2010; Kosalka 2012).[15] Placing the onus on Muslim or minority groups perpetuates myths that have re-emerged in the past decade in Canada (and elsewhere) as part of a growing discontent with multiculturalism (Ryan 2010), evident in critiques of religious and cultural difference and in a resurgence of an "us versus them" discourse (e.g., Beaman 2012-13).

David Mitchell, a fourteen-year-old Ontario student, gave the *Globe and Mail* (Mitchell 2010) a telling account of when and how the topic of sex came up when he was with his friends, admitting that more often than not they talked about video games without anyone "suddenly announcing" facts about sex or sexuality. Mitchell further discussed access to the Internet, describing the time he was dared to enter "blue waffle" into Google and subsequently discovered what a particular sexually transmitted disease looks like. Beyond Mitchell's story, however, students were not provided space to respond to the proposed changes or even to comment on whether they were aware of the media firestorm. After McGuinty announced his decision to halt the proposed changes, the teachers' unions posted statements on their websites regarding the curriculum, but students were not provided with the same space to voice any reflections.

The Final Decision: A Diverse Province

In response to the swift controversy over the curriculum, Premier McGuinty backed away from the policy changes:

> The fact of the matter is that we have a very diverse province. And I think that it's very important that as a government when we develop policies of any kind – but especially when it comes to sex education in our schools, something that touches our children directly – that we listen very carefully to what parents have to say and we take their concerns into account and lend shape to a curriculum that they are comfortable with.[16] (*CBC News* 2010c)

In response to the final decision by the Ontario government, Malcolm stated that he gave God the glory and that the decision was "a victory for the Canadian children" (*CBC News* 2010c). McVety went further, stating, "It is unconscionable to teach eight-year-old children same-sex marriage, sexual orientation and gender identity ... It is even more absurd to subject sixth graders to instruction on the pleasures of masturbation, vaginal lubrication, and 12-year-olds to lessons on oral sex and anal intercourse" (ibid.).

Topics pertaining to sexuality and sexual identity should be discussed in the home, but dismissing the importance of addressing these topics in the classroom is very problematic. That students can and will learn about sex from peers, online, or through other sources does not diminish the responsibility to educate them (accurately) in the classroom. They can also learn about world history through Wikipedia, yet no one seems to feel that this source is a valid replacement for history classes in the education system.

The responses of groups such as the Institute for Canadian Values and Canada Christian College repeat and reaffirm a problematic assumption about religious identity and ideology when discussing sexual diversity: that religious individuals necessarily stand in opposition to sexuality, sexual diversity, or discussions of sexuality in the classroom. As McGarry (2008) argues, this approach constructs the queer subject as a quintessentially secular subject.[17] Further, it does not allow room in the public arena for religious voices that do not stand in opposition to sex education, let alone those whose identity encompasses being both religious and a sexual minority.

I, along with others (both in this volume and elsewhere), challenge the notion of this fundamental clash between religion and sexuality. It is evidenced repeatedly that we move fluidly across boundaries of identity, yet it is often seen as "normal" for opposition to sexual diversity to be based on religious ideologies. I am not suggesting that there is unequivocal support among the "nonreligious" for anyone who is sexually different; even when sexual diversity is seemingly embraced, there is still a normative standard regarding sexuality, which a number of scholars (e.g., Duggan and Hunter 2006; Valverde 2006; Cossman 2007; Denike 2007, 2010) argue simply reshapes heternormativity into a standard of homonormativity.

Reflecting on Identity: Religion and Sexuality

I have outlined debates from the 2010 controversy over the sex education curriculum in Ontario to illuminate how media and public discourses about religion and sexual difference frame them as necessarily in opposition. These standards and stereotypes perpetuate misconceptions of identity regarding religion and sex or gender and allow for essentialist ideas about identity. Narrow frameworks and narrative scripts posit religion as "naturally" in opposition to teaching about sex and healthy sexuality. The dominant narrative of normative religious identity versus non-normative sexual identity has been based on a particular mainstream construction and supported as "natural" in public institutions. To what extent do anxieties about sexuality and sexual orientation and the assumption that the religious will necessarily be at odds with them frame what we are willing to teach or what we expect students to learn?

Earlier in the chapter, I asked: if we are teaching about sex and sexuality, what are we also teaching about religion and religious ideology? It seems fairly clear that the expectation of opposition to teaching about sex, sexual acts, sexuality, and sexual orientation is based on the implication that a certain advocacy will be undertaken if these topics are raised in the classroom. That is, teaching about sexuality or sexual orientation becomes framed as advocating alternative lifestyles. We therefore teach that religion is somehow intolerant of sexual diversity (regardless of whether this assumption is true) and end up making both religion and (normative) sexuality into single and essentialized constructs. The proposed curriculum for sex education, which outlines any number of body parts, acts, and identity aspects, was reframed – not only by individuals such as McVety and Malcolm but also by some of the parents questioned – so that what students would be taught was understood as instructions on how to perform various sexual acts and how to question one's sexual identity.

Even though the curriculum speaks of "gender identity and sexual orientation," it is quite clear that it was not the normative identities or orientations that were causing the controversy – no one expressed concern that teachers would discuss heterosexuality or model heternormativity. Rather, the language circled around an implicit agenda: worry about the supposed "conversion" of heterosexual, gender-normative youth into non-normative "others." The use of the "slippery slope" argument, here and in other debates about gender and sexual difference, presupposes that by addressing a topic such as sexual orientation, "naturally" heterosexual youth will be converted to homosexuality. As McKay stated, students were already aware of the fact of sexual difference when entering a classroom; the curriculum includes the topic in order to provide factual information on the subject as a way of dispelling misconceptions regarding sexual difference (Nguyen 2010).

The assumed conflict between religion and sexuality also demonstrates arguments made by numerous scholars on the relationship between religion and secularity. "Social and political agendas and institutions construct 'religion' in different times and places in relation to other equally unstable concepts such as secular and profane" (Goldenberg, forthcoming). Changes in religious ideologies, which become embedded in a set of legislative or policy doctrine in response to public or cultural demands, demonstrate the ways that social agendas construct the place and role of religion at any given time. Jakobsen and Pellegrini (2008, 1) ask, "How did it come to pass that secularism as a 'world' discourse was also intertwined with one particular religion?" They argue that the secularism narrative mistakenly posits secularism as a universal trait somehow different from particularized religion when, in fact, "secularism remains tied to a particular religion, just as the secular calendar remains tied to Christianity" (ibid., 3). Jakobsen and Pellegrini critique the commonly held assumption that secularism and secularity are the binary opposite of religious ideologies. As they explain,

> Our argument is not that this secularism is really (essentially) religion in disguise, but rather that in its dominant, market-based incarnation it constitutes a specifically Protestant form of secularism. The claim of the secularization narrative is that the secularism that develops from these European and Christian origins is, in fact, universal and fully separate from Christianity. (Ibid.)

Although it would be tempting to point only to the politics of McGuinty's decision or to the politics of media reporting, there is another factor to be considered: who responds most vocally to these discussions in the media and why? The role of moderate organizations needs to be considered. I have argued that "selling" the story often involves polarizing views and sensationalizing voices; but it is also the responsibility of moderate organizations and voices to communicate their perspectives.

As the media articles outlined above demonstrate, there is an intrinsic, often combative relationship between sexuality and religion, which is repeated and reperformed through social and legal standards and through a discourse that permits the framing of sexual difference and religious beliefs as incompatible. It is almost paradoxical that at a time when Canada's tolerance toward diversity was under scrutiny (Ibbitson 2011), we found ourselves with a province that, when faced with opposition to discussion regarding healthy sexuality, gender identity, and sexual orientation, halted proposed changes that had taken two years to develop.

Queering Spaces?

In the 2010 controversy over the sex education curriculum in Ontario, the space of the debates remained focused on the "religious" opposition to the topics it introduced. As a result, the curriculum has retained its heteronormative foundations, and students such as David Mitchell will still be expected to rely on nonschooling sources of information for sexual education beyond these foundations. The declaration of ownership of the school by external sources, influences, and voices successfully framed the debates about the sex education curriculum, allowing these voices to dominate in the public sphere. This dominance created confusion about what the revisions entailed, and it silenced, or at least distracted from, the voices of the policy makers who had worked on the changes, the administrators who were to oversee them, the teachers who were to implement them, and the students who were to receive the proposed education.

Oswin (2008) explores the use of sexuality in the production of space, namely how geographies of heternormativity are reproduced in such areas as housing initiatives, family planning programs, and migration policies. Perhaps the way to connect identities lies in the use of queer theoretical approaches regarding identity, such as Oswin's work on queer geographies, Jakobsen and Pellegrini's (2008) critique of secular discourse and queer identities, and Denike's (2007, 2010) arguments regarding the normalizing processes used for the sexually different. Incorporating the tools of queer theory exposes the assumed static nature of identity, leaving room for the dynamic means by which individuals live across the boundaries of their identities at any time. Using the education system to convey that gender identity and sexual orientation are both given and diverse, not subjects of controversy, could possibly open up new dialogues about the way that sex, gender, and sexuality are discussed both at a public level and in media.

This chapter brings together diverse theoretical approaches to examining the construction of religious identity markers in relation to discussions about sexuality to critique the supposedly unified, static nature of these categories of identity and to demonstrate the fluidity with which we cross and mesh boundaries of identity and difference. I am interested in thinking through the ways that we connect these identities. Rather than continuing to portray and perpetuate identity categories as incompatible in public discourse, it seems imperative to challenge the misuse of identity categories in order to develop ways to discuss sex, gender, and sexuality within an educational context that do not result in what has been witnessed in the Ontario case: the removal of sexual acts, sexual bodies, and sexual orientation – in short, the removal of sex – from sex education.

Notes

I would like to thank all the participants at the workshop held at Queen's University in preparation of this volume, who offered insightful critiques of an early version of this chapter. I would also like to thank two anonymous reviewers for UBC Press, who made suggestions for revision, resulting in a clearer essay and argument.

1 For further analysis, see Valaitis (2011), who argues that the "proposed revisions to the Ontario sex education curriculum failed to gain public support because of the Government's inability to adequately prepare for and mediate the Province's competing liberal and conservative sexual ideologies" (ibid., ii).
2 To be clear, I am not suggesting that the groups identified in this chapter as being opposed to the proposed curriculum changes are representative of all religious viewpoints on this subject or of religiosity in general. Part of what I am interested in challenging is how some religious views become constructed and accepted as "the" religious view – which I argue here, and elsewhere (Shipley, forthcoming), does a disservice to a wide spectrum of religious groups and individuals who do not share the same views.
3 Lisa Reimer taught music at Little Flower Academy, a Catholic high school for girls in Vancouver. When she originally signed the one-year contract, she accepted a clause indicating that as a non-Catholic she would not speak out against the Catholic faith or try to sway students toward non-Catholic values. Reimer told the school administration of her sexual orientation when she requested parental leave in December 2009 because her partner was expecting a baby. She was denied leave and subsequently told to stop teaching in the classroom in response to parental complaints about having a lesbian teach their children (*CBC News* 2010a).
4 Analysis of public versus private spaces regarding identity politics is beyond the scope of this chapter, although I note here that often in these debates arguments centre on what is or is not "allowable" in public versus private spaces.
5 This contextualization of religious doctrine can be evidenced in numerous ways, including the creation of queer-friendly religious organizations, as well as interviews regarding individual practice and identification. For discussion of the ways that queer religious women live their identities in Los Angeles, see Wilcox (2010).
6 To be clear, I am not proposing that we poll students about the content of their education, but if we are to understand "what students should learn," it does seem germane to know whether they feel the sex education curriculum is in any way relevant or helpful for them as they develop. One response, by student David Mitchell, is mentioned later in this chapter. Formally, however, the debate has centred on what certain religious groups have stated and on brief interviews with parents.
7 Dalton McGuinty resigned in October 2012, one year after securing his third win in a provincial election. In February 2013 Kathleen Wynne was sworn in as premier. She has stated that she will bring the sex education curriculum back to the table.

8 Experts asked to contribute to the changes have argued that teaching young children the proper names for genitalia can, among other benefits, help them to identify potential sexually inappropriate behaviours (Sex Information and Education Council of Canada n.d.).
9 Anyone who has attempted to purchase clothes for females under the age of ten will have noticed the increasing range of miniskirts and halter tops available for female children; for some reason, this is less offensive than the possibility of teaching children the words "penis," "vagina," or "testicle."
10 This focus is demonstrated by the titles of related news articles, such as "Religious Groups Fight Changes to Ontario Sex Ed Curriculum" (*Maclean's* 2010), and by media statements like "Religious groups objected to the revised curriculum" (*CBC News* 2010c).
11 Hammer and Howlett (2010b) also state that when it comes to sex education "almost every change or revision ... has drawn some objections" since it was first introduced in Ontario in 1966.
12 Salaam Canada is a queer Muslim community. For more information, see http://salaamcanada.org.
13 The list of interveners in the 2004 *Reference Re Same-Sex Marriage* decision in Canada included religious groups in support of same-sex marriage in Canada, such as the United Church of Canada and the Liberal Rabbis in Support of Same-Sex Marriage. Although the reference stated that religious officials would not be required to marry same-sex couples if they were opposed, it is evident that not all religious groups or individuals felt concern about doing so.
14 Canada has experienced several controversies regarding religion, minority practices, concepts of multiculturalism, and views on accommodation. For more details, see Ibbitson (2011).
15 The *National Post* stated that although the strongest resistance was from religious groups, their presence in the debate "should not distract thoughtful secularists from the fact that the program is objectionable on purely rational grounds," given that between early childhood and adolescence, children's imaginations are not naturally attuned to sex (McParland 2010).
16 Following the original writing of this chapter, Dalton McGuinty introduced an anti-bullying policy, the Accepting Schools Act (Government of Ontario 2012), which prohibits bullying based on sexual orientation, gender, disability, race, religion, and other grounds. The policy outlines, among other things, that all publicly funded institutions (which includes Catholic schools in Ontario) are required to allow student clubs that foster gay-straight alliances – the subject of much consternation from a new coalition of religious organizations.
17 In other studies, including Molly McGarry's work in this instance, reference to the queer subject pertains specifically to sexual difference. In contrast, the example here

of "the" religious response to the Ontario sex education curriculum broadens the queer subject to include anyone who is willing to publicly discuss topics of genitalia, healthy sexuality, and understanding bodies.

References

Amsterdam, A.G., and J. Bruner. 2000. *Minding the Law: How Courts Rely on Storytelling, and How Their Stories Change the Ways We Understand the Law – and Ourselves*. Boston: Harvard University Press.

Beaman, L. 2012-13. Battles over Symbols: The "Religion" of the Minority versus the "Culture" of the Majority. *Journal of Law and Religion* 28 (1): 101-38.

Benzie, R. 2010. Analysis: Dalton McGuinty's Sex-Ed Surrender Motivated by Politics. *Toronto Star*, 23 April. http://www.thestar.com/news/ontario/2010/04/23/analysis_dalton_mcguintys_sexed_surrender_motivated_by_politics.html.

Beyer, P. 2008. From Far and Wide: Canadian Religious and Cultural Diversity in Global/Local Context. In *Religion and Diversity in Canada*, ed. L. Beaman and P. Beyer, 9-39. Leiden: Brill.

Burn, S.M. 1996. *The Social Psychology of Gender*. San Francisco: McGraw-Hill.

Butler, J. 1993. *Bodies That Matter: On the Discursive Limits of "Sex."* New York: Routledge.

CBC News. 2010a. Lesbian Teacher Told to Work from Home, Group Says. 28 April. http://www.cbc.ca/news/canada/british-columbia/lesbian-teacher-told-to-work-from-home-group-says-1.871199.

–. 2010b. McGuinty Supports New Sex Ed Curriculum. 20 April. http://www.cbc.ca/news/canada/toronto/mcguinty-supports-new-sex-ed-curriculum-1.948362.

–. 2010c. Sex Ed Opponents Claim Victory in Ontario. 23 April. http://www.cbc.ca/news/canada/toronto/sex-ed-opponents-claim-victory-in-ontario-1.899830.

Cossman, B. 2007. *Sexual Citizens: The Legal and Cultural Regulation of Sex and Belonging*. Stanford, CA: Stanford University Press.

Denike, M. 2007. Religion, Rights, and Relationships: The Dream of Relational Equality. *Hypatia* 22 (1): 71-91.

–. 2010. Homonormative Collusions and the Subject of Rights: Reading Terrorist Assemblages. *Feminist Legal Studies* 18 (1): 85-100.

Dickey Young, P. 2008. Two By Two: Religion, Sexuality and Diversity in Canada. In *Religion and Diversity in Canada*, ed. L. Beaman and P. Beyer, 85-104. Leiden: Brill.

Duggan, L., and N.D. Hunter. 2006. *Sex Wars: Sexual Dissent and Political Culture*. New York and London: Routledge.

Foucault, M. 1978. *The History of Sexuality*. Vol. 1, *An Introduction*. Trans. R. Hurley. New York: Random House.

–. 1985. *The History of Sexuality*. Vol. 2, *The Use of Pleasure*. Trans. R. Hurley. New York: Vintage.

–. 1988. *The History of Sexuality.* Vol. 3, *The Care of the Self.* Trans. R. Hurley. New York: Vintage.

Gleason, M. 1999. *Normalizing the Ideal: Psychology, Schooling, and the Family in Postwar Canada.* Toronto: University of Toronto Press.

Goldenberg, N.R. Forthcoming. Queer Theory Meets Critical Religion: Are We Starting to Think Yet? In *Theories of Religion,* ed. R. King. London: Routledge.

Government of Alberta. 2009. *Bill 44: Human Rights, Citizenship and Multiculturalism Amendment Act.* http://www.assembly.ab.ca/ISYS/LADDAR_files/docs/bills/bill/legislature_27/session_2/20090210_bill-044.pdf

Government of Ontario. 2012. *Bill 13: Accepting Schools Act.* http://ontla.on.ca/web/bills/bills_detail.do?locale=en&BillID=2549.

Hammer, K., and K. Howlett. 2010a. Muslims, Christians Challenge Ontario's More Explicit Sex Ed. *Globe and Mail,* 21 April. http://www.theglobeandmail.com/news/politics/muslims-christians-challenge-ontarios-more-explicit-sex-ed/article1542657.

–. 2010b. Ontario to Introduce More Explicit Sex Education in Schools. *Globe and Mail,* 20 April. http://www.theglobeandmail.com/news/national/ontario-to-introduce-more-explicit-sex-education-in-schools/article4315814.

Howlett, K., and K. Hammer. 2010. Ontario Salvages Reworked Curriculum, Minus the Sex Part. *Globe and Mail,* 27 April. http://www.theglobeandmail.com/news/national/ontario-salvages-reworked-curriculum-minus-the-sex-part/article4316752.

Ibbitson, J. 2011. Kirpan Ban Puts Canada on Brink of Multiculturalism Debate No One Wants. *Globe and Mail,* 11 February. http://www.theglobeandmail.com/news/politics/ottawa-notebook/kirpan-ban-puts-canada-on-brink-of-multiculturalism-debate-no-one-wants/article611650.

Jakobsen, J.R., and A. Pellegrini, eds. 2008. *Secularisms.* Durham, NC: Duke University Press.

Kinsey, A. 1998a. *Sexual Behavior in the Human Female.* 1953. Reprint. Bloomington, IN: Indiana University Press.

–. 1998b. *Sexual Behavior in the Human Male.* 1948. Reprint. Bloomington, IN: Indiana University Press.

Knott, K. 2009. From Locality to Location and Back Again: A Spatial Journey in the Study of Religion. *Religion* 39 (2): 153-84.

Kosalka, P. 2012. Religious Persecution in Canada. 16 April. http://www.theinterim.com/issues/society-culture/religious-persecution-in-canada/.

Maclean's. 2010. Religious Groups Fight Changes to Ontario Sex Ed Curriculum. 22 April. http://www2.macleans.ca/2010/04/22/religious-groups-fight-changes-to-ontario-sex-ed-curriculum.

McGarry, M. 2008. "The Quick, the Dead, and the Yet Unborn": Untimely Sexualities and Secular Hauntings. In *Secularisms,* ed. J.R. Jakobsen and A. Pellegrini, 247-79. Durham, NC: Duke University Press.

McGuire, M.B. 2008. *Lived Religion: Faith and Practice in Everyday Life*. Oxford: Oxford University Press.

McParland, K. 2010. Explicit Sex Education Program Planned for Ontario. *National Post*, 21 April. http://fullcomment.nationalpost.com/2010/04/21/national-post-editorial-board-explicit-sex-education-program-planned-for-ontario.

Mitchell, David. 2010. YouTube: The REAL New Sex Ed Curriculum. *Globe and Mail*, 27 April. http://www.globecampus.ca/blogs/family-view/2010/04/27/youtube-real-new-sex-ed-curriculum.

Nguyen, L. 2010. Ontario Premier Defends Sex-Ed Curriculum. *National Post*, 20 April. http://www.whale.to/b/sex67.html.

Ontario Ministry of Education. 1998. *The Ontario Curriculum, Grades 1-8: Health and Physical Education*. http://www.edu.gov.on.ca/eng/curriculum/elementary/health.html.

Oswin, N. 2008. Critical Geographies and the Uses of Sexuality: Deconstructing Queer Space. *Progress in Human Geography* 32 (1): 89-103.

Rayside, D. 2010. Sex Ed in Ontario: Religious Mobilization and Socio-Cultural Anxiety. Paper presented at the Annual Meeting of the Canadian Political Science Association, Concordia University, Montreal, Quebec, June. http://www.cpsa-acsp.ca/papers-2010/Rayside.pdf.

Reference re Same-Sex Marriage. 2004. 3 S.C.R. 698, S.C.C. 79.

Ryan, P. 2010. *Multicultiphobia*. Toronto: University of Toronto Press.

Schippert, C. 2005. Queer Theory and the Study of Religion. *Revista de Estudos da Religião* 5 (4): 90-99.

Sex Information and Education Council of Canada. n.d. http://www.sieccan.org.

Shipley, H. Forthcoming. Religious and Sexual Orientation Intersections in Education and Media: A Canadian Perspective. *Sexualities and Religion*, in press.

Suh, E.M. 2002. Culture, Identity Consistency, and Subjective Well-Being. *Journal of Personality and Social Psychology* 83 (6): 1378-91.

Valaitis, V. 2011. "Righting" Sex-Ed in Ontario: Adult Anxiety over Child and Adolescent Sexual Knowledge and the Government's Undemocratic Mismanagement of Ideological Pluralism. MA thesis, Queen's University. http://hdl.handle.net/1974/6544.

Valverde, M. 2006. A New Entity in the History of Sexuality: The Respectable Same-Sex Couple. *Feminist Studies* 32 (1): 155-62.

Wilcox, M. 2010. *Queer Women and Religious Individualism*. Bloomington: Indiana University Press.

Winnubst, S. 2006. *Queering Freedom*. Bloomington: Indiana University Press.

5

When Religion Meets Sexuality
TWO TALES OF INTERSECTION
Andrew Kam-Tuck Yip

For many nonreligious people in secular liberal democracies such as the United Kingdom, religion is widely perceived as a constraining and restrictive force, antithetical to a contemporary society that values personal liberty, difference, pluralism, and diversity. In my view, this perception is most evidently manifested in contestations about gendered and sexual bodily subjectivities, performances, and practices, such as the controversy surrounding religious dress codes (e.g., the veil), sexual equality legislation (e.g., parenting rights for same-sex couples), and sex education in schools (e.g., the proposed curriculum in Ontario; see Shipley, Chapter 4, this volume). From this perspective, the intersection of religion and sexuality necessarily leads to tension and conflict, manifested in individuals' deference to religious institutional and community diktats, exacting high psychological and social costs for those who do not fall within the rigid and narrow definition of acceptable sexual and gender expression, namely (heterosexual) sex only within marriage. Therefore, it often baffles nonreligious people why any individual, particularly the young, would choose to align with an institutional space that seems to curb the full expression of one's humanity. This is of course a simplistic and exaggerated account of the intricate relationship between religion and sexuality, underscored by the "secularism-democracy-choice" ideological nexus. Although there is undeniably an empirical basis to this discourse, there is also another tale to be told, which presents a more positive outcome, encapsulating voices of integration and accommodation.

Within this context, this chapter aims to present my broad reflections on the intersection between religion and sexuality. My reflections are based on empirical data drawn from various research projects on, generally, lesbian, gay, and bisexual (LGB) Christians, Muslims, and Buddhists, as well as on heterosexual and LGB religious young adults of diverse religious faiths. Whereas some chapters in this volume focus on broader political and cultural processes embroiled in the debate on sexual and religious pluralism, this chapter's spotlight is on religious social actors' diverse experiences in managing such tensions in everyday life and on their social and political implications. Although the research on which this chapter is based was undertaken in the United Kingdom, the broad theme on the intersection of sexuality and religion is also relevant to the study of LGB people with religious faith in Canada as social actors who endeavour to construct integrated sexual and religious identities by engaging with different enabling and constraining factors.[1]

I would like to emphasize two more points at this stage. First, the corpus of empirical data from which I draw focuses primarily on Christianity and Islam. Bearing in mind that there are inter- and intrareligious similarities and differences across religions, any attempt to essentialize and generalize religion should be discouraged. This is particularly crucial if we are committed to a "lived religion" or "everyday religion" perspective that prioritizes the multifaceted lived experience and the agentic capacity of religious actors rather than the institutional dimension of religious teachings and praxis (e.g., Ammerman 2007; McGuire 2008). Second, the two broad tales this chapter presents should not be considered exhaustive, static, and mutually exclusive. As will become clear, these tales could represent a trajectory or a journey from a space of tension and conflict to one of integration and growth. Often, this process is conceived as a journey of spiritual growth, where one matures in one's relationship with oneself, others, and the divine. There could be a host of factors that facilitate this process, such as access to, and consumption of, online and offline social and theological support (e.g., support networks and LGB-affirming popular and scholarly sexual theology). From a sociological and psychological perspective, this process could be seen as the development of a positive identity, often leading to a heightened politicization of religious faith and sexuality, as well as to better social adjustment. This is not to say that the journey is unidirectional. Rather, it has the potential to take different twists and turns, making the management of tension and conflict and the development of integration very much an everyday experience and practice of religious and sexual actors.

The First Tale: Tension and Conflict

The uncomfortable and awkward relationship between sexuality and Christianity is widely documented in scholarly literature. This interaction is well summarized by Hunt (2010, xi):

> Sexuality ... has long been a matter of taboo for the Christian Church, remaining marginalized, even ostracized, rarely discussed in polite ecclesiastical circles. Above all, its sensual, provocative and unpredictable nature, particularly when expressed through fornication, adultery and homosexuality – hedged in by prohibitions inherited from its Judaic origins – has endured as an anathema to Christian spirituality and the ethos of Christ-like purity.

Structuring this Christian construction of sexuality is the dualistic conception of the human: with the mind and the body as polar opposites. One is supposed to train the mind, which directs bodily performances, to focus its gaze on the divine, the transcendent, the nonphysical – in other words, everything that sanctifies and makes one close to holiness. The mind, therefore, is closely associated with the spiritual and the sacred. In contrast, the body is constructed as a repository of corrupted and corrupting desires that could distract one from what is pure or, worse, tempt one to sin through unacceptable bodily performances. The body, therefore, represents the profane. It is a vehicle that could lead one to sinfulness; thus its desires must be controlled by the mind (e.g., Ellingson and Green 2002; Yip 2010b).

Admittedly, this characterization is broad and general. Nonetheless, it underpins the diktat of sex only within marriage that the Christian Church generally upholds. Furthermore, empirical research continues to show that the management of bodily desires and performances, particularly those of a sexual nature, continues to preoccupy much of the Christian Church and its believers. For instance, Sharma (e.g., 2008, 2011), in her study of primarily heterosexual young women in conservative Protestantism, has shown that her participants were constantly aware of the dominant sexual discourse of appropriate or respectable female sexuality, generating much conflict in their lives, as the discourse does not reflect the diverse ways that they understood and practised their sexuality. Therefore, there was a gap between the dominant sexual discourse and lived experiences. This tension, of course, exists not only among Christian religious actors. Scholars have shown that it is also present in other religious faiths (e.g., Machacek and Wilcox 2003; Morgan and Lawton 2007).

This dominant discourse of sexuality polices sexual desires and expressions, executing surveillance on religious actors' subjectivity and behaviour, significantly through the web of institutional and interpersonal power relations. The internalization of religious norms – at times strengthened by cultural norms – that legitimize and perpetuate heteronormativity also leads to self-policing that complements institutional and social policing. Often, this self-policing is made even more potent by the recognition of an omnipotent, omniscient, and omnipresent divine power (e.g., God), who is discursively constructed as the origin and guardian of such heteronormative norms and values. This multilayered surveillance and policing produces a "panoptic gaze" from which no one can escape. Thus one feels that one is constantly being watched and judged, which creates the need to be "proper" or "respectable," mindful of the costs of transgressing orthodox sexual and gender orders (Foucault 1977, 1979). Of course, religious believers, as social actors, are not cultural dupes who conform to such norms uncritically. Reponses to such a "panoptic gaze" are diverse, a point that is emphasized throughout this chapter. Indeed, this disciplinary power could generate outcomes that extend beyond social control and regulation because "under certain conditions, disciplinary power may expand the possibilities of the self" (Green 2010, 331).

However, in this section, I focus on the theme of tension and conflict, which is prominent in all the projects this chapter covers. Undoubtedly, this theme represents a significant lived reality for religious actors who depart from the injunction of sex only within marriage, heterosexual and nonheterosexual alike. These experiences and voices are documented in the project Religion, Youth and Sexuality.[2] For instance, only 59.5 percent of self-identified heterosexual participants claimed to "agree" or "strongly agree" that "my religion is positive towards sexuality."[3] Among participants who self-identified as "lesbian," "gay," "homosexual," or "bisexual," the percentage was noticeably lower at 36.8 percent.[4] In addition, only

39.3 percent of heterosexual participants[5] – and 34.9 percent of non-heterosexual participants[6] – claimed to "agree" or "strongly agree" that "my religion understands the issues lesbian, gay and bisexual people face."

The qualitative data of this project offers us a closer look at the challenges that this scenario presents. A good example of this is the story of Jodie, an orthodox Jewish bisexual woman, who repeatedly narrated stories about the tension and conflict theme in the interview and the video diary. She went to great lengths to reduce such tension, first by terminating a same-sex relationship and then by toeing the official line, as it were, by plunging herself into a cross-sex relationship only to discover that there were also many challenges in relation to intimacy, sexuality, and religious faith. Her narrative, recorded over a week, has been organized as follows to enhance continuity and to illustrate the prominence of this struggle in her life:

> I am bisexual, and my decision [is] that I want to actively try to limit myself to dating only men because I can't see myself living [in] a long-term relationship with a woman because of my community and my religion ... I started having a relationship with a girl, and then at some point during the relationship, I admitted to myself that I was gay. [But] I didn't feel comfortable being Orthodox Jewish and gay, in that I don't want to live in a fringe community. So my choices were: leave orthodoxy and embrace myself as gay ... or break off the relationship and embrace my orthodoxy ... If you are homosexual and still want to actively identify as Jewish, then you are pretty much part of a fringe group ... I couldn't leave Orthodox Judaism. That was my home, my people, where I feel comfortable. I was willing to give up a good relationship that I had been in for two years ... [Referring to her current cross-sex relationship where the partner self-identified as Jewish and gay] I am more attracted to girls and he is more attracted to boys, so how do we really know that we are interested in each other? It is a difficult call, so we decided to be physical in our relationship ... [Initially,] I had clear limits. I would go so far as kissing and perhaps some feeling, exploration, but I draw the line at mutual masturbation and any sort of penetrative, oral or anal sex ... [But] in the past week there has definitely been some oral sex and ejaculation and that is a bit confusing to me, and I presume it is confusing him in the same way ... If you were to ask me straight out if it is allowed or

forbidden, I would say forbidden. But I did it and didn't feel emotionally bad afterwards. Emotionally, I feel great about that because it means that I can keep doing what comes naturally without having to feel stressed about it. But mentally, I am a bit worried about that.

This narrative clearly illustrates Jodie's experience of tension and conflict, precipitated by her keen desire to belong to an ethnic and religious community that gave her an ontological anchor in life. However, this belonging, as she acknowledged, had strings attached. She was painfully aware of the heterosexist nature of the community's requirements regarding her emotional attachment and bodily performances, which made her same-sex relationship unsustainable. And she was concerned about observing the requirement of sex only within marriage, which filled her with a sense of guilt and shame about her heterosexual relationship. On both fronts, she felt that she had failed to live up to the religious and ethnic ideal of a "proper" relationship.

Interestingly, research has shown that religious actors have varied understandings of what constitutes "sex." In contrast to Jodie, some draw a firm line between vaginal penetration as "real" or "full" sex and other sexual acts as tolerable – or at least less unacceptable – experimentation (e.g., Johansson 2007; Regnerus 2007; Freitas 2008). Some of the single heterosexual participants in the project Religion, Youth and Sexuality deployed this rationalization. Tariq, a heterosexual Muslim man, firmly drew a line of demarcation between vaginal penetrative sex (i.e. "full sex"), which he considered wrong outside of marriage, and other types of sexual activity that were deemed less "sinful." This line of demarcation at least partly informed his decision not to have a long-term relationship. Therefore, for the time being, he limited himself to recreational sex that he rationalized as not "full" or "real" sex. This strategy helped him to reduce the tension between his bodily desire and his commitment to religious injunction:

> Obviously, I have done things with girls, but I have never actually had sex ... I have never actually had full sex ... Oral, like blow jobs and other things, which I have had ... but I have never had penetrative sex because that is a boundary which I cannot cross, because I know it is another sin I am committing. I am committing a sin indulging in oral

sex, etc., but I don't want to go to the higher platform of penetrating a girl. [*Interviewer:* It is more sinful outside of a marriage?] Yeah. If you are married, you are a one-person girl or one-person guy ... [Oral sex] is not sex ... I have refrained from getting into relationships, and I like being single ... because if I got into a serious relationship, I am going to have [full] sex ... It would be wrong ... If I end up having penetrative sex and it doesn't work out between me and the girl, then I have sinned ... I can't have [full] sex, yeah, because it is against my religion. The thing is that I want sex, but in the middle is a whole battlefield. So I am always in conflicting emotions ... I think if I wasn't Muslim, I would be sexually active on a regular basis. But because I see the context of Islam and the reasons why they don't want you to be sexually active as such, I see it as more pure and more holy, etc. So ... I do refrain myself ... It is a battlefield of emotions and thoughts that I am in a constant struggle with ... So it is a balance I have to personally find.

Among LGB religious actors, one of the most commonly deployed strategies to reduce tension and conflict is to compartmentalize their religious faith and sexuality. This strategy involves a conscious effort to conceal their sexual orientation in heteronormative spaces such as a place of worship or the family, where they know being open about their sexual orientation could potentially exact a high cost. Thus sexuality is deliberately downplayed in such spaces, and religiosity is sometimes heightened to overcompensate for sexuality. The presentation of the heterosexual self (i.e., acting the heterosexual role) is therefore crucial in this context, at least in signposting one's ability to conform to heteronormative religious and cultural norms such as marriage.

In contrast, in spaces that are deemed safe, LGB religious actors foreground their sexuality, and their religious identity then assumes a secondary position. Interestingly, these safe spaces, including the LGB community, could be inhospitable to those who profess a religious faith due to the anti-religion undercurrents of such spaces, which arise from the connection between LGB identity and secularity in the dominant discourse of LGB identity construction. The following comments by Muhammad, a gay Muslim, illustrate that such a strategy of compartmentalization is multifaceted:

> I think until I can confidently tell everybody that I am gay and Muslim, two in one, I will have to, you know, in a way, lie about who I really am ... Except my sister, nobody at home and in my extended family knows I am gay. What they see is a nice Muslim boy, and one day I will get married and stuff, have children, you know, I will be respectable in the community ... So I play along really, being a nice Muslim boy. People just assume I am heterosexual but not ready for marriage yet. But when I am in the gay scene, some people laugh when I tell them I am Muslim. They don't seem to understand why this South Asian gay boy wants [to have something] to do with Islam ... I think Islamophobia is rife in the gay scene, just like in the society. So [when I am] there, I am just gay, and an exotic Asian boy, [and] my religion is thrown out of the window ... It is rather one-dimensional, don't you think?[7]

In the same vein, Alyson, a self-defined "queer" Christian woman, also talked about this kind of experience in multiple entries in the video diary she kept for the project Religion, Youth and Sexuality, arranged as follows to enhance continuity and flow:

> I suppose I've grown up compartmentalizing bits of my life ... because I just divide things into compartments like my girlfriends and my parents, they don't meet ... And in some ways, my gay friends and [straight friends] ... At one point I was in the Catholic students' group ... Catholic Students' Society and the LGBT Society, and I had these two completely [separate] sets of friends and they never met. And I'm quite good at that and I don't think it is necessarily a good thing ... For ten years I was keeping bits of my life completely separate ... I had a queer life, I had a queer community ... and for a year I moved back with my parents ... But where we live, there is not really any kind of gay community, and I think that in some ways I really, really miss that. Just having the assumption that not everyone here is straight ... And anyway, it was just this very isolated experience really, and I think in some ways that had made me realize that actually I do want these parts of my life to be connected together, and for things to be less disjointed and less isolated and less compartmentalized.

Muhammad's and Alyson's narratives demonstrate intricate presentations of the self in diverse spaces. Their own norms, requiring appropriate bodily performances and vocabulary, informed how they positioned themselves in the interactional web. As they intended, this positioning was crucial to the social meanings that others attached to some aspects of their self.

In addition to the compartmentalization strategy, a host of other strategies have been documented in LGB religious actors' management of tension and conflict. One strategy is to suppress sexuality in order not to undermine belonging to a religious community, which often means opting for abstinence. Some go even further and attempt "healing" with spiritual intervention in order to lead a "normal" life of heterosexuality. Another strategy is to leave religious spaces and forgo religious pursuits altogether. In these cases, sexuality and religious faith become mutually exclusive. A third strategy is to embark on a journey to locate and construct LGB-friendly religious and spiritual spaces that allow sexuality and religious faith to flourish (e.g., Kubicek et al. 2009; Browne, Munt, and Yip 2010).

The Second Tale: Integration

The above section has focused on the experiences of heterosexual and LGB religious actors in managing the tension and conflict generated by the ideal of sex only within marriage, which also carries a heterosexist undertone. In this section, the spotlight is turned on three categories of religious actors who relate to this ideal in different ways, all of whom are largely comfortable with the integration of religious faith and sexuality in their lives. Of course, as I have mentioned, this does not mean that they no longer experience tension in their sexual and spiritual journeys since new decisions need to be made and old decisions are subjected to re-evaluation in this ongoing process of constructing a meaningful life.

The first of these categories comprises heterosexual religious actors who are committed to the ideal of sex only within marriage and who refrain from any sexual activity until marriage, thus "saving themselves for marriage." Quantitative data from the project Religion, Youth and Sexuality show that 76.1 percent of the heterosexual participants who were single did not consider themselves "sexually active."[8] As I have shown above, there were different understandings about what "sex" and "being sexually active" meant. Nonetheless, qualitative data show that some participants were indeed committed to not having any kind of sexual activity outside of marriage. Samarah, a heterosexual Muslim woman, asserted her commitment to this ideal:

> [Being a heterosexual woman means] ... just like getting married to a man, I'm going to get married ... Because in my religion you are not allowed to have relationships outside of marriage, and you are only allowed to have relationships to the person you are married to ... I do think it is wrong to do that, to have different partners, or just to have sex before marriage, because you should only have one partner ... I would say the point of getting married is to know them intimately and if you know them like that before getting married, what would be the point of getting married?

In addition, 39.5 percent of heterosexual participants who were in an unmarried partnered relationship did not define themselves as "sexually active."[9] Layla, a heterosexual Muslim woman who was in a relationship, also decided to refrain from engaging in any sexual activity. She talked to her partner about not wanting to kiss, let alone to go any further, but was fully aware of the challenge this would entail:

> I'm not going to lie, it [abstaining from sex in a relationship] does [prove to be challenging]. But then at the end of the day, there is a goal [marriage] that you're working towards that just helps dull it. It's another challenge, but yes you just have to deal with it ... We actually had that talk [about kissing]. In my head I'm saying probably no, but then again as the situation arises I told him you never know what the moment is. It's not like you're going to switch on in your brain, no don't kiss him, as this moment arises ... I wouldn't say I'm the best Muslim in the world because I still learn every day ... But the little that I do know, I will stick firmly to that, so I am not going to compromise my beliefs for this relationship ... He actually said that that was one of the reasons that attracted him to me ... because he's been looking for that kind of girl for a while ... I'm definitely not having sex until marriage ... To me I believe it [sexual pleasure within marriage] will actually be ten times more because you're with someone that you waited for.

It is tempting to interpret the narratives above as evidence that religious faith put constraints on the participants in the management of their sexual desires and bodily performances. This reading would fit into a taken-for-granted yet pervasive secular discourse that constructs religion as necessarily sex-negative, or at least sex-constraining. If pushed too far, this discourse could frame the decision making illustrated by Samarah and Layla as ill-informed, even irrational and nonagentic. I contend that such an interpretation is inaccurate because it does not recognize the agency of the social actors concerned: their capacity to construct values and practices regarding their sexuality that draw from their religious faith as a primary source. In fact, such decisions could be a reflection of self-expression and self-actualization in the effort to construct a meaningful and integrated life. A parallel debate can be found among the views of scholars and commentators on Muslim women who wear the veil to consciously demonstrate religious and/or political piety and/or to defy popular discourse that constructs the veil as a symbol of gender oppression and as anathema to liberty and choice (e.g., Gehrke-White 2006; Ahmed 2011).

The second category of heterosexual religious actors comprises those who are emotionally committed to marriage as an appropriate rite of passage in their lives but who, for various reasons, are not in the position to marry due to, for instance, the unavailability of a suitable partner. For those already in a relationship, the reason might be that the right time for marriage has not yet arrived due to, say, a lack of financial and/or occupational security. In the Religion, Youth and Sexuality study, these religious actors explained that they engaged in sexual activity within the context of the relationship without developing a sense of failure over not conforming to the ideal of sex only within marriage. A case in point was Martin, who defined himself as Christian-Muslim but did not define his sexuality. He was in a cohabiting, heterosexual, unmarried relationship against the religiously informed wishes of his and his partner's parents. He rationalized the situation as follows:

> Me and my fiancée we are not married ... we live together, and obviously we do have sexual relations, which my mum's religion [Christianity] would condemn, and so would Islam ... The reason we don't get married is because we want to have good jobs, and we want everything to be sorted out and marry afterwards and be secure. We do feel that we are married. We do everything together, I cook, I help ... it's like I'm living a married life ... Even though the religion says that you shouldn't [have sex] before

marriage, we think that we are more than married, and so as long as we are happy with each other, and we are not forcing on each other ... And so we do live like a married couple ... Obviously, we are very cautious and, you know, I would not get her pregnant ... and she wouldn't try to do that, to upset the family. So I think we have a very good relationship as a couple, and we know that when it comes, it comes ... and we will be able to have kids and everything will be fine ... Our god is a god of love, so He does understand, and we are not doing something that is just sex. And I think that comforts us ... So till we get married we just kind of save [money] and build our lives ... We are pretty much in love, and from the three years I know her, nothing really changed. My feelings never changed.

In this account, Marcus evoked qualities that characterize a religiously sanctioned relationship, such as love, care, commitment, and faithfulness, even though these qualities were not experienced within the context of a marriage – as yet. Although he acknowledged the tension that others' lack of affirmation of their living arrangement might entail, he and his fiancée were able to reconcile their religious commitment and sexual and emotional needs in their marriage-like relationship. He acknowledged the religious and cultural ideal as a part of their future sexual and religious biographical narratives and, indeed, as an appropriate stage in their life course, one embedded in their future planning (for more details, see Page, Yip, and Keenan 2012). However, as far as the present was concerned, their departure from the ideal was rationalized to minimize tension. This strategy demonstrates the individualization of sexual ethics, where sexual bodily performances that fall outside the remit of the ideal are constructed as progressing toward a future that will eventually embrace the ideal.

Stories of Transgression and Transformation
The third category of religious actors within this "integration" theme refers specifically to those who identify as "lesbian," "gay," or "bisexual."[10] Compared to their heterosexual counterparts, who benefit from heteronormativity, LGB religious actors occupy a unique position within the dominant religious discourse of sexuality. More often than not, they are, to use a term that Collins (1986) deploys within the context of race and gender in reference to black women, "outsiders within": gendered and

sexual bodies that are out of place and experientially disconnected from the gender and sexual orders. Specifically, they are outsiders within a space that in principle includes them on the basis of religious faith, but the incompatibility between their counternormative sexuality and the heteronormative sexual and gender orders militates against the development of a complete and consistent sense of "insiderness." This intricate insider-cum-outsider status can exact high psychological and social costs in terms of identity integration and interpersonal relationships, at times leading to "moving out of the space" as a strategy to reduce or resolve conflict. Stories of conflict, alienation, and fear told by LGB actors across religious faiths are well documented in academic and nonacademic literature (e.g., Browne, Munt, and Yip 2010; Yip, Keenan, and Page 2011; Yip and Page 2013). I have also covered them to a certain extent in the first empirical theme of this chapter.

Here, I would like to focus on stories that are less audible and present in dominant scholarly and popular discourses. These are stories about transgression and transformation that offer hope and optimism. I must emphasize that we should not essentialize such stories. They are dynamic and emergent, often coming out of – and building upon – stories of conflict, alienation, and fear. They are voices that were once banished to the marginal space – silenced even – but that are gradually being mainstreamed into the discourse of religious principles and praxis. The marginal space is no doubt a space of oppression and alienation, but it also contains the seed of productive and transformative energy. The following comments by Jemimah, a lesbian Muslim, powerfully demonstrate this aspect of marginal space:

> I think there are particular gifts that come by being in a sexual minority and having to remake your spirituality outside of the mainstream of a faith. I think the gift in that is that we have to learn to love and to practise our faith in a different way, and we have to consider what purpose creation might have in having created us. I think there is always a gift in being marginalized and that gift is always a way of transforming the notion of identity altogether into something higher, it's actually to transcend stuff ... We experience exclusion both in the way scripture is understood and expounded and in the way that religious worship and faith practice is actually set up. There is no blueprint for our participation

in those things, and sometimes we are excluded or executed or eliminated explicitly and sometimes implicitly. And that is the story of queer sexuality anyway in society at large, [so] why should it be any different in religion? It's more acute in religion because people think they've got the word of God behind them.[11]

A paradigmatic and epistemological shift takes place when LGB religious actors, having learned to trust their own positive lived experiences, turn shame and guilt into pride and courage, unleashing an emancipatory energy that liberates and transforms not only their own lives but also the institutional and cultural underpinnings of the religious space. From the Simmelian perspective of the "stranger," this shift represents an intricate balance in the union between closeness/involvement (i.e., attachment to, desire for, full membership) and remoteness/indifference (i.e., lack of access to full membership). This balance offers a simultaneously near and far positionality that generates a criticality and a political sensibility that together transform a religious actor's relationship with the self (i.e., one learns to accept sexuality as a legitimate part of personhood and humanity), with others (i.e., one learns to relate to others as an integrated person), and with God/the divine (i.e., one learns to believe that sexuality does not precipitate God's rejection).

Therefore, on the personal level, sexuality is no longer a sinful appendage of one's personhood but the core of one's spiritual self, a means to connect, relate, and unite with oneself, others, and God/the divine truthfully and honestly. In other words, sexuality and spirituality coalesce in one's personhood, spiritual path, and social relationships (for more details, see Yip 2005b). Indeed, the transformation of shame into pride, as Munt (2007, 3-4) reminds us, could lead to psychic, political, and cultural realignment and empowerment:

> Shame is peculiarly intrapsychic: it exceeds the bodily vessel of its containments – groups that are shamed contain individuals who internalise the stigma of shame into the tapestry of their lives, each reproduce discrete, shamed subjectivities, all with their own specific pathologies ... Shame has a compound materiality, including a compound mentality, and its effects therefore can be unpredictable. Shame is also an emotion

that can flow unrecognisably through the subject, it can saturate a person and s/he may yet remain oblivious to its results, merely experiencing a diffuse unyielding sadness ... Shame has political potential as it can provoke a separation between the social convention demarcated within hegemonic ideals, enabling a re-inscription of social intelligibility. The outcome of this can be radical, instigating social, political and cultural agency amongst the formerly disenfranchised.

Such transformation also applies to the spiritual dimension. Once this transformation is achieved, scriptural verses such as the following take on new and inclusive meanings of connection and acceptance to which an LGB religious actor can relate:

> God, *you* fashioned me in my mother's womb ... For I am awesomely and wondrously made. (Psalms 139: 13-14, emphasis added)

> O people, We created you all from a male and female and made you into *different* communities and *different* tribes, so that you should come to know one another, acknowledging that the most noble among you is the one most aware of God. (Qur'an 49: 13, emphasis added)

This transformation of shame into pride is not limited to the personal level. Indeed, LGB politics and scholarship within religious spaces – with support from their heterosexual counterparts in some cases, as well as with interreligious and religious-secular collaboration – have transformed theology as well as institutional culture and praxis. Space here does not allow for a detailed discussion of such scholarship, but this transgressive corpus of work, particularly on Christianity, is increasingly compelling religious actors and religious authorities to re-examine fundamental issues such as how theology ought to be done and how God ought to be conceived, with the aim of grounding conceptions of the divine in lived experiences, contemporary knowledge, and socio-cultural realities (for a detailed analysis of such scholarship on various religious faiths, see Yip 2010a).

On a political level, LGB religious actors – having trusted the integration of their religious faith and sexuality and decided to embody this integration in everyday life – directly and indirectly assert a difference of salient spiritual significance in the acquisition of sexual rights. The concept of "sexual citizenship" or "intimate citizenship" is useful in theorizing their effort in this respect. Sexual/intimate citizenship emphasizes the rights to practice/conduct, identity, and relationship without discrimination, regardless of sexual and gender identities (Richardson 2000a, 2000b; Plummer 2003). Within the British context, this discourse is increasingly well established in the secular sphere, particularly in light of the expansion of sexual equality and human rights legislation with the enactment of the Equality Act of 2010, which establishes "sexual orientation" as a "protected characteristic" (Government of the United Kingdom 2010). Thus sexual rights are linked inextricably to civil, social, and political rights to which every citizen is entitled. As Oleksy (2009, 4) explains,

> Intimate citizenship theory describes how our private decisions and practices have become intertwined with public institutions and state policies, such as public discourse on sexuality, legal codes, medical system, family policy, and the media ... Processes appearing at the overlap of the public and the private realms have an immense impact on the redefinition of the concept of citizenship ... A broad approach to the concept of citizenship makes it clear that it is no longer possible to theorize citizenship in universal and abstract terms, but that it should always be situated in the context of an individual lived experience. Seen from this perspective, citizenship's territory must be extended beyond the conventional public sphere and, consequently, located at the intersection of many axes of social, political, and cultural stratification ... It is impossible to interpret and articulate citizenship without always situating it in a lived experience.

Admittedly, such social, political, and legal progress has not been as evident in religious spaces, demonstrated by religious institutions' repeated attempts to seek exemption from sexual equality legislation on the basis of religious conscience. Such attempts have mainly been unsuccessful (see also Jakobsen, Chapter 1, this volume). There is no denying that religiously motivated homophobia and biphobia are still rife in religious spaces. Nonetheless, equality and human rights discourses from the secular sphere are infiltrating the religious sphere, evidenced by the discursive shift from LGB rights to human rights. If one's humanity is part and parcel of the created order, then exercising one's right to live a full life, including sexual life, is not merely a sexual matter but also a religious matter and indeed a human and citizen matter. If stratification within broader society on the basis of sexual orientation is untenable, unethical, and indeed illegal, the religious sphere cannot be insulated from this development even though it continues to perpetuate such stratification. LGB religious actors who, despite all the risks and costs, have chosen to remain within the religious sphere could bring about this move toward human rights. They are emboldened by an ontological security that is firmly anchored in God or the divine, who understands their oppression and will deliver them from this plight. Therefore, the social and political capital that they construct is buttressed by "spiritual capital," part of which is the belief that the quest for sexual justice is inalienable from the broad quest for social justice because God is justice. Such endeavours are often characterized by a desire to return to the essence of religious faith, its broad principles and norms, as opposed to institutional rules.

Some may consider this view of the transformative potential of the marginal space to be overly optimistic given the incontrovertible rise of increasingly media-savvy and financially secure anti-LGB politics in religious and secular spaces (e.g., Sullivan-Blum 2009; Viefhues-Bailey 2010). I acknowledge that the battle of sexual politics is far from over, particularly within religious spaces. However, I also think that there is incontrovertible evidence of progressive developments within religious and secular spaces that are a reason for optimism and an impetus for future work.

Concluding Remarks

This chapter has highlighted two primary manifestations of the intersection of religion and sexuality. Using the themes of "tension and conflict" and "integration," informed by various empirical research projects, I have shown that, although varying degrees of tension and conflict are indeed a lived reality for many religious actors, their management strategies are diverse. In this respect, there is evidence that some heterosexual and LGB religious actors individualize sexual ethics not only to reduce tension and conflict but also to integrate various aspects of their lives. Their understandings of, and relationships with, the diktat of sex only within marriage is therefore multilayered. Objective, institutional, and externally imposed norms are often reinterpreted, being informed by subjective, positive, personal experiences and individualized approaches to ethical behaviour in sexual bodily performances.

In the case of LGB religious actors, the intersection of religion and sexuality can also spark transformative energies that challenge the cultural ideology of heteronormativity. Essentially, such stories are about the reorientation of identity: the sick and unacceptable sinner is transformed into the wholesome human being who has been created and blessed by God and is worthy of equal rights. This is an important epistemological shift because it liberates LGB religious actors from constructing subjectivities and bodily performances in line with negative social definitions. This shift enables them to develop positive and proud self-definition and self-expression. As Wetherell (2010, 4) reminds us, "Identity continues to be the place where collective action, social movements, and issues of inequality, rights and social justice come into focus and demand attention." Indeed, the political dimension of this identity is salient, reminiscent of identity politics of other kinds that are used to transform oppression into liberation in individual and collective life:

> Historically, identity politics has had both an activist and an academic existence. Activists involved in successful social movements, such as the civil rights movement and the women's movement, who self-consciously invoked the concept of identity in their struggles for social justice held at least the following two beliefs: (1) that identities are often resources of knowledge especially relevant for social change, and that (2) oppressed groups need to be at the forefront of their own liberation. (Alcoff and Mohanty 2006, 2)

In the case of LGB religious actors, this identity politics is more than a human political strategy for resistance and change. It also has salient spiritual significance and symbolism because of the belief that God is on their side as a god who delivers people from oppression, in line with the divine vision of justice, inclusivity, and fairness. This belief that God and other significant religious figures (e.g., Jesus and Muhammad) are on their side significantly emboldens their spirit, strengthens their resilience, and expands their individual and collective agency for change.

Notes

1 Indeed, a parallel project, Religion, Gender and Sexuality among Youth in Canada, which makes use of the questions used in the UK study Religion, Youth and Sexuality: A Multi-faith Exploration (Yip and Page 2013), is presently underway in Canada (see http://www.queensu.ca/religion/Faculty/research/dickeyyoung.html).
2 The project Religion, Youth and Sexuality: A Multi-faith Exploration (Yip, Keenan, and Page 2011; Yip and Page 2013) was funded in the United Kingdom by the Arts and Humanities Research Council and by the Economic and Social Research Council under the Religion and Society program. The research team consisted of Andrew Kam-Tuck Yip (principal investigator), Michael Keenan (co-investigator), and Sarah-Jane Page (research fellow). The project, conducted between 2009 and 2011, involved 693 participants, each of whom completed an online questionnaire. In addition, 61 participants were interviewed, and a further 24 completed a week-long video diary. The participants, aged between eighteen and twenty-five, were drawn from six religious faiths. More details of the project can be found at http://www.nottingham.ac.uk/sociology/rys. The research team is grateful for the funding, as well as for the invaluable contribution of the participants, the individuals and groups who helped to recruit the sample, and the members of the advisory committee (see also Yip and Page 2013; and Keenan, Yip, and Page, forthcoming).
3 The valid responses totalled 421.
4 The valid responses totalled 106.
5 The valid responses totalled 415.
6 The valid responses totalled 106.
7 This quotation is from my primarily qualitative project A Minority within a Minority: British Non-heterosexual Muslims, conducted in 2001-02 (see Yip 2004, 2005a). Twenty female and twenty-two male participants completed a brief questionnaire and were interviewed individually. In addition, two focus group interviews (one mixed and one all-women) were held. I gratefully acknowledge the financial support of the Economic and Social Research Council in the United Kingdom and the important contribution of all participants and user groups.
8 The valid responses totalled 331.
9 Some participants who were in this type of relationship defined themselves as nonheterosexual (e.g., as "bisexual"). The valid responses to the question totalled 153.
10 It must be acknowledged that although I use the term "LGB," the discussion focuses on lesbians and gay men primarily. Undoubtedly, there are significant similarities between these three groups, but the politics surrounding bisexuality often takes on a different dimension in the discourse of sexual rights and sexual morality. Bisexuals, for instance, are often subjected to greater pressure to opt for heterosexuality, compared to their lesbian and gay counterparts, because they supposedly have such a choice. Further, they are often erroneously considered incapable of monogamy in a coupled relationship because of the perception that they need to have partners of

different sexes simultaneously. Misunderstandings such as these have led to the stigmatization of bisexuals within heterosexual, as well as lesbian and gay, communities (e.g., Toft 2009).

11 This quotation is from the Queer Spiritual Spaces project (Browne, Munt, and Yip 2010), conducted in 2008-09, which was funded in the United Kingdom by the Economic and Social Research Council. Sally Munt was the principal investigator, and Andrew Yip and Kath Browne were the research advisers, partly supervising the research fellows.

References

Ahmed, L. 2011. *A Quiet Revolution: The Veil's Resurgence, from the Middle East to America*. London: Yale University Press.

Alcoff, L., and S. Mohanty. 2006. Reconsidering Identity Politics: An Introduction. In *Identity Politics Reconsidered*, ed. L. Alcoff, M. Hames-García, S. Mohanty, and P. Moya, 1-9. Basingstoke, UK: Palgrave.

Ammerman, N.T. 2007. *Everyday Religion: Observing Modern Religious Lives*. Oxford: Oxford University Press.

Browne, K., S.R. Munt, and A.K.T. Yip, eds. 2010. *Queer Spiritual Spaces: Sexuality and Sacred Places*. Farnham, UK: Ashgate.

Collins, P.H. 1986. Learning from the Outsider Within: The Sociological Significance of Black Feminist Thought. *Social Problems* 33 (6): 175-93.

Ellingson, S., and M.C. Green, eds. 2002. *Religion and Sexuality in Cross-Cultural Perspective*. London: Routledge.

Foucault, M. 1977. *Discipline and Punish: The Birth of the Prison*. Harmondsworth, UK: Penguin.

–. 1979. *The History of Sexuality*. Vol. 1, *An Introduction*. Harmondsworth, UK: Penguin.

Freitas, D. 2008. *Sex and the Soul: Juggling Sexuality, Spirituality, Romance, and Religion on America's College Campuses*. Oxford: Oxford University Press.

Gehrke-White, D. 2006. *The Face behind the Veil: The Extraordinary Lives of Muslim Women in America*. New York: Citadel.

Government of the United Kingdom. 2010. *Equality Act*. http://www.legislation.gov.uk/ukpga/2010/15/contents.

Green, A.I. 2010. Remembering Foucault: Queer Theory and Disciplinary Power. *Sexualities* 13 (3): 316-37.

Hunt, S., ed. 2010. *The Library of Essays on Sexuality and Religion: Christianity*. Farnham, UK: Ashgate.

Johansson, T. 2007. *The Transformation of Sexuality: Gender and Identity in Contemporary Youth Culture*. Aldershot, UK: Ashgate.

Keenan, M., A.K.T. Yip, and S. Page. Forthcoming. Exploring Sexuality and Religion Using an Online Questionnaire. In *How to Research Religion: Putting Methods into Practice*, ed. L. Woodhead. Oxford: Oxford University Press.

Kubicek, K., B. McDavitt, J. Carpineto, G. Weiss, E.F. Iverson, and M. Kipke. 2009. "God made me gay for a reason": Young Men Who Have Sex with Men's Resiliency in Resolving Internalized Homophobia from Religious Sources. *Journal of Adolescent Research* 24 (5): 601-33.

Machacek, D.W., and M.M. Wilcox. 2003. *Sexuality and the World's Religions*. Santa Barbara, CA: ABC-Clio.

McGuire, M.B. 2008. *Lived Religion: Faith and Practice in Everyday Life*. Oxford: Oxford University Press.

Morgan, P., and C.A. Lawton. 2007. *Ethical Issues in Six Religious Traditions*. Edinburgh, UK: Edinburgh University Press.

Munt, S.R. 2007. *Queer Attachments: The Cultural Politics of Shame*. Aldershot, UK: Ashgate.

Oleksy, E.H. 2009. Citizenship Revisited. In *Intimate Citizenships: Gender, Sexualities, Politics*, ed. E.H. Oleksy, 1-16. London: Routledge.

Page, S., A.K.T. Yip, and M. Keenan. 2012. Risk and the Imagined Future. In *Ashgate Research Companion to Religion and Sexuality*, ed. S. Hunt and A.K.T. Yip, 255-70. Farnham, UK: Ashgate.

Plummer, K. 2003. *Intimate Citizenship: Private Decisions and Public Dialogues*. Seattle: University of Washington Press.

Regnerus, M.D. 2007. *Forbidden Fruit: Sex and Religion in the Lives of American Teenagers*. Oxford: Oxford University Press.

Richardson, D. 2000a. Constructing Sexual Citizenship. *Critical Social Policy* 20 (1): 105-35.

–. 2000b. *Rethinking Sexuality*. London: Sage.

Sharma, S. 2008. Young Women, Sexuality and Protestant Church Community: Oppression or Empowerment? *European Journal of Women's Studies* 15 (4): 345-59.

–. 2011. *Good Girls, Good Sex: Women Talk about Church and Sexuality*. Winnipeg: Fernwood.

Sullivan-Blum, C.R. 2009. "It's Adam and Eve, not Adam and Steve": What's at Stake in the Construction of Contemporary American Christian Homophobia. In *Homophobias: Lust and Loathing across Time and Space*, ed. D.A.B. Murray, 48-63. Durham, NC: Duke University Press.

Toft, A. 2009. Bisexual Christians: The Life-Stories of a Marginalised Community. In *Contemporary Christianity and LGBT Sexualities*, ed. S.J. Hunt, 67-85. Aldershot, UK: Ashgate.

Viefhues-Bailey, L.H. 2010. *Between a Man and a Woman? Why Conservatives Oppose Same-Sex Marriage*. New York: Columbia University Press.

Wetherell, M. 2010. The Fields of Identity Studies. In *The Sage Handbook of Identities*, ed. M. Wetherell and C.T. Mohanty, 3-26. London: Sage.

Yip, A.K.T. 2004. Negotiating Space with Family and Kin in Identity Construction: The Narratives of British Non-heterosexual Muslims. *Sociological Review* 52 (3): 336-50.

–. 2005a. Queering Religious Texts: An Exploration of British Non-heterosexual Christians' and Muslims' Strategy of Constructing Sexuality-affirming Hermeneutics. *Sociology* 39 (1): 47-65.

–. 2005b. Religion and the Politics of Spirituality/Sexuality. *Fieldwork in Religion* 1 (3): 271-89.

–. 2010a. Coming Home from the Wilderness. In *Queer Spiritual Spaces: Sexuality and Sacred Places,* ed. K. Browne, S.R. Munt, and A.K.T. Yip, 35-50. Farnham, UK: Ashgate.

–. 2010b. Sexuality and Religion/Spirituality. *Sexualities* 13 (6): 667-70.

Yip, A.K.T., M. Keenan, and S. Page. 2011. *Religion, Youth and Sexuality: Selected Key Findings from a Multi-faith Exploration.* Nottingham, UK: University of Nottingham Press.

Yip, A.K.T., and S. Page. 2013. *Religious and Sexual Identities: A Multi-faith Exploration of Young Adults.* Farnham, UK: Ashgate.

6

Women, Sex, and the Catholic Church
THE IMPLICATIONS OF DOMESTIC VIOLENCE FOR REPRODUCTIVE CHOICE

Catherine Holtmann

Women's sexuality has long been a flashpoint in the history of Christianity, and issues related to women's sexuality have increasingly come to divide contemporary Catholics. This is certainly the case in the Canadian Catholic Church, where women experience the paradoxes of their religion. Catholic women in Canada are subjects under civil law yet are often treated as objects according to church teachings. Canadian Catholic bishops have condemned intimate-partner violence yet remain silent about sexual violence more generally, including situations in which women are pregnant. Church leaders publicly promote the dignity of human persons and their "right to life" but do not acknowledge women's rights when it comes to their own bodies. Priests are aware of the legitimacy of divorce in cases of domestic violence, but some continue to promote a rhetoric of Catholic family life that does not include important information about the reality of abuse and violence. Although it might be argued that many Catholics have left the church as a result of the secularization of contemporary society, it can also be argued that some have left as a result of these paradoxes. There is little space within the church's institutional structures for women to engage with these profoundly social and deeply religious issues. For many Catholics who choose to remain within the church, it has become an uncomfortable place. Often parish life is a site of conflict or has been made pious and impersonal in efforts to avoid controversy.

This chapter describes some aspects of the contemporary situation of women and sexuality from the perspectives of Catholics themselves, based on social science data collected from well over a hundred Canadian Catholics, most of whom live in Atlantic Canada. The analysis is situated within the context of sociological theorizing on women and religion as well as within the context of Catholic social teachings. The women reflexively interpret the Catholic Church's principles of social justice in light of their lived experiences at the nexus of sexuality, reproductive choice, and domestic violence.

Catholicism is a global religion – what happens in any part of the church has a potential ripple effect. At the Second Vatican Council, the church defined itself as the people of God *and* as hierarchical (Flannery 1988). This has resulted in complex dynamics in terms of authority and change, particularly since women are the majority of active Catholics (D'Antonio et al. 2001; Pew Research Center 2008) yet are excluded from ordained ministry. Women's inability to formally participate in decision making in diocesan, national, and international structures certainly presents them with challenges; however, it also offers them opportunities in terms of imaginatively engaging with the richness of the tradition.

Women are among the poorest people in society, shouldering the primary responsibility of caring for children, the ill, and the elderly (World March of Women 2000; United Nations 2010). They carry out the vital work of ensuring human survival while comprising the majority of the victims of intimate-partner violence, rape, and armed conflict (United Nations 2008). Women are confronted with the effects of incredible social and environmental problems that put their daily lives at risk. This is the context in which women manage their sexual identities and make reproductive choices utilizing a variety of resources, including their Catholic faith. Along with chapters by Andrew Kam-Tuck Yip, Donald Boisvert, Nancy Nason-Clark, and Heather Shipley in this volume, my research highlights how religion is both a valuable and problematic resource in the challenging work done at the junctures of religion and sexuality.

Sociological Research on Religion

Scholars of religion suggest that in globalized society religion helps to establish personal identity and contribute to the social order (Van Pelt Campbell 2007). Ammerman (2003) theorizes that coherence in religious identity is constructed continually in relationships of social solidarity. Religious identity is constructed simultaneously on individual and social levels. Particularly when considering patriarchal religious groups, it is important to understand how women's religious agency is embedded within religious structures that outsiders may consider oppressive (Mahmood 2001; Korteweg 2008). All women find themselves within a matrix of power relationships; religious women are not simply victims in a system without power. In the midst of the problematic experiences of their lives, they are capable of managing multiple identities by bringing together aspects of what have been understood traditionally as secular and sacred worldviews (Nason-Clark and Fisher-Townsend 2005). Catholic women exercise religious agency in complex ways. Sometimes this agency appears unambiguously religious, such as when they pray or proclaim readings from scripture during mass. At other times women's actions may appear outwardly secular but be guided by religious convictions, such as when they advocate on behalf of the poor or make reproductive choices in intimate relationships.

In Chapter 1 of this volume, Jakobsen describes the complexity of moral agency in Foucauldian terms, noting that individual sexual *freedom* in the United States is highly *regulated* within the overarching social discourses of political biopower and economic free markets. Utilizing the discourse of freedom, both government agencies and transnational corporations actively slot citizens into sexual hierarchies based on race, class, gender, and sexual orientation. Jakobsen asserts that gay, lesbian, and queer people can exercise moral agency in resisting heteronormative discourses that oppress them.[1] Agency, be it moral and/or religious, personal and/or collective, is always influenced by cultural discourses and institutions. Exercising agency is about reflexively considering intersecting discourses and making strategic choices (Archer 2007). Persons, groups, and institutions undergo change through social interactions. Catholic women's embodiment and sexuality are lived experiences that are dynamic, being situated at the intersection of androcentric laws, roles, relationships, and responsibilities articulated by Catholic leaders, by biblical examples of nonjudgmental compassion for the suffering, and by a profit-driven economy in which women's bodies are commodified by cosmetic, fashion, and entertainment industries. They exercise religious agency in self-identifying as Catholic while making reproductive choices and supporting others to do the same in a context where these choices are often impacted by at least the threat, if not the reality, of abuse and violence in intimate relationships (see Nason-Clark, Chapter 9, this volume).

In her work on lived religion, McGuire (2008) exposes the historical construction of boundaries between the sacred and the secular that took place in the history of western Europe. The distinctions between what is presently considered properly religious and what is not are social constructions, the results of human struggles over cultural resources and power. Boundaries that are used to determine what constitutes legitimate religion have been contested over time. McGuire asks sociologists to reconsider the sacred-secular dichotomy by focusing on the everyday practices of people and the meanings that people themselves give to these practices. This theoretical emphasis on lived religion has propelled my sociological research on women and religion toward the margins of institutional life. Similar to Shipley's contribution in Chapter 4 of this volume, my work explores the perceptions, conceptions, and lived spaces with which Catholic women manage the secular and religious values of choice and life.

Sociological studies of Catholics in North America point out the variety of ways that members live the paradoxes of their church. Research on Catholic women's religious orders in the United States and Canada has shown that despite the drastic decline in numbers, these women have used their resources in the service of faith-based social action for the common good (Ebaugh 1993; Wittberg 1994, 2006; Gervais 2012). Whereas Wittberg (1994) maintains that social action is the key to the renewal of vowed religious life for Catholic women, Ebaugh (1993) asserts that women's religious orders have lost their primary purpose. She argues that Catholic women no longer need exclusive female communities in order to fulfil their aspirations for participation in social change because the feminist movement has ensured that all women, regardless of the form of their religiosity, can participate in public life. In line with the historical ministry and self-understanding of women in religious orders, married Catholic women with increased access to rich theological resources are claiming the religiosity of their sexual relationships and choices as women in the church.

Winter, Lumis, and Stokes (1995) have found that Christian women, from the conservative to the progressive, employ the strategy of "defecting in place" to manage their feelings of religious alienation. Catholic women, because of their longstanding exclusion from ordained ministry, sometimes choose to form women-church communities in order to self-educate, exercise leadership, and celebrate a distinct religiosity. These communities began in the 1980s as spaces for feminist theological consciousness raising and spiritual practice. They do not exclude women's participation in Catholic parish structures (Radford Ruether 1986). One aspect of this religiosity is a heightened sensitivity to women's experience of social inequality (Holtmann 2008b). Experiences of religious alienation have become a foundation for working for justice on behalf of others – a central principle of feminist praxis since one's knowledge of oppression and one's action for change can reciprocally inform each other (Hartsock 1998). Wallace's (1992) research shows that Catholic lay women have not only formed women-church spaces but have also exercised pastoral leadership at the parish level due to a shortage of ordained clergy.

Other studies of women's involvement in parish life further reveal the diversity of leadership cultures within Catholic parishes and diocesan structures, some of which are more favourable to women's leadership but all of which are tenuously dependent on benevolent clergy attitudes (Bouclin 2006; Howard Ecklund 2006; Ternier-Gommers 2007). In her study of pro-change Catholic movements, Dillon (1999) claims that identities are constructed within the context of special-interest groups that are explicitly Catholic by using interpretations of doctrine and scripture that support progressive views. Canadian examples of Catholic women's pro-change organizations include the French-based L'autre Parole and Femmes et ministères (Couture 2008) and the English-based Catholic Network for Women's Equality (CNWE) (Dunne 2008). The CNWE was formed in 1981 in Canada and is part of a network of Catholic pro-change groups that includes the Women's Ordination Conference and the Women-Church Convergence in the United States, the We Are Church movement in Europe, and the international organization Women's Ordination Worldwide.

Despite some degree of commonality among progressive and conservative Catholics in terms of core practices, symbols, and values (D'Antonio et al. 2001; D'Antonio and Pogorelc 2007), the contradictions between Catholic women's commitment to social justice for women and the problematic exercise of their agency within institutional structures are contributing to what Baggett (2009, 175-76) refers to as "civic underachieving" and "civic silencing" among Catholics as a whole. The Catholic hierarchy's censure of theologians, clerics, and nuns who support increased opportunities for women's leadership and decision making in the church has resulted in increased conflict and polarization within the church (Holtmann

2011). An example of this is the Congregation for the Doctrine of the Faith's (2012) assessment of the Leadership Conference of Women Religious (LCWR) in the United States. The assessment condemned the LCWR's doctrinal errors concerning issues of women's ordination, the correct pastoral care of homosexual persons, and certain "radical feminist themes." Polarization and conflict among Catholics in regard to social justice for women prevent critical debates about a gendered approach to Catholic social teachings that could incorporate a complex understanding of women's sexuality and reproductive choices in a context of pervasive violence against women.

Catholic Social Teachings
Social action on the basis of faith has a place in the modern Catholic Church. At least since the late nineteenth century, Catholic leaders have written public documents outlining the church's teachings on critical social issues. Catholic laity have been encouraged to read the signs of the times, acknowledging the profound spiritual relationship between the church and the world (Flannery 1988). In their daily lives, Catholics are called to engage in the task of a global movement toward a more just social order that respects the dignity of the individual as well as the common good. Included in the "signs of the times" identified by Catholic leaders in the 1960s were the dignity and rights of women in domestic and public life (Beattie 2010). In a sociological analysis of the Second Vatican Council, Wilde (2007) shows how its progressive theological outcomes were largely a result of the organizational strategies of the voting participants. Many bishops were convinced that Catholics around the world should address and contribute to amelioration of the problems caused by social inequalities. However, although issues of concern to Catholic women regarding sexuality and reproductive choice were known to the bishops, they were not on the agenda for change. Following the Second Vatican Council, the papal encyclical *Humanae Vitae* of 1968 firmly cemented the Catholic hierarchy's position against birth control, despite substantial dissent (Radford Ruether 2006). The Vatican continues to oppose public sex education, artificial birth control, and abortion. Nevertheless, surveys indicate that 80 percent of sexually active American Catholic women who regularly attend mass use contraception and that 85 percent approve of abortion when a woman's health is seriously endangered (Catholics for Choice 2014).

Popes John Paul II (1995) and Benedict XVI (2009) promoted the "feminine genius" of women in their roles as wives and mothers and in their responsibility for the protection of life from conception to grave. Pope Francis is also doctrinally conservative (Squires 2013). The precariousness of women's sexual lives is never realistically considered. Nevertheless, some national bishops' conferences have attempted to address further issues of concern to women (Canadian Conference of Catholic Bishops 2000).

Catholic social teachings are structural in their approach to the analysis of social problems, critiquing the ways that political and economic institutions deepen societal inequalities and contribute to human suffering. Yet for the most part, they fail to include a realistic analysis of social power in the process of change. It is exceedingly difficult to change entrenched power dynamics, and attempts to do so often expose institutionalized violence (Pfeil 2008). Issues regarding women and sexual ethics were only slowly conceptualized as public social problems and were usually relegated to the private sphere (Hunt 2005). This treatment of such issues is evidence of the androcentric nature of Catholic social teachings, where women's input, based on their experiences of domination, has been practically absent (Beattie 2010). Traditional Catholic theology maintains a dualistic anthropology that considers men and women to be complementary – that is, equal in dignity yet different in their essential human natures. Descriptions of complementary sexual relationships are highly idealized, and despite acknowledging the general oppression of women, they neither fully appreciate the prevalence of intimate-partner violence, particularly when women seek to alter relational dynamics in marriage, nor draw connections to sexism and essentialist conceptualizations.[2]

Having condemned many forms of violence, including terrorism, the Vatican has not explicitly acknowledged spousal violence or sexual violence against women in marriage, the family, or war (Pontifical Council for Justice and Peace 2005). Canadian bishops, however, have issued two public statements, including one from the Social Affairs Commission of the Assembly of Quebec Bishops entitled *A Heritage of Violence: A Pastoral Reflection on Conjugal Violence* (1989). The Quebec bishops acknowledge the pervasiveness of conjugal violence, which includes psychological, verbal, physical, sexual, and institutional forms of violence. They admit that aspects of the church's history and practice may have contributed to the abuse of women by their husbands, including the patriarchal nature of Christianity, the church's overemphasis on women's roles as wives and mothers, the exclusively masculine nature of liturgical language, the exclusion of women from sacramental ministry, and the overemphasis on marriage "for better or for worse" (ibid. 1989). The second statement, from the Canadian Conference of Catholic Bishops (CCCB), entitled "To Live without Fear" (2000, 73), refers to violence against women as a "sin, crime and serious social problem." The CCCB affirms the work of the Quebec bishops and encourages Catholics to work with others in society for short- and long-term solutions. These pastoral statements were issued just prior to Statistics Canada's release of the results of the National Violence against Women Survey, which showed that 29 percent of Canadian women aged eighteen or older had experienced at least one act of physical or sexual violence committed by their current or former spouse (Johnson and Dawson 2010, 67).

Many Canadian bishops, like their counterparts around the world, have become increasingly vocal in the public sphere about their anti-abortion stance in all circumstances, including rape (Canadian Press 2010). This is the case despite a historical tradition of permitting abortions in certain circumstances (Maguire 1984). Unlike the religious reasoning that led to a theory of just war, which never dares to single out soldiers for committing moral crimes, there has been little attempt by Catholic leaders to consider the moral complexity involved in the reproductive choices that women encounter when they live in a context where violence is more pervasive than it is in war. The unequivocal pronouncements from Rome and elsewhere against reproductive choice deny Catholic women moral and religious agency in the very arena for which they are supposedly specialized due to their essential nature.[3] The CCCB established the Catholic Organization for Life and Family in the mid-1990s, yet none of its publications refer to domestic violence (COLF 2013). Have Canadian bishops forgotten their public condemnation of domestic violence (Holtmann 2013)? Sexual assault (attempted or actual forced sexual contact or intercourse) is the most underreported crime in Canada. Its prevalence is suspected to be high given that women are most likely to be assaulted by someone they know (Johnson and Dawson 2010, 94). The bishops' silence about sexual and intimate-partner violence is of concern to Catholics for whom social justice is a "constitutive dimension" of the gospel (Gunn and Lambton 1999). Many have interpreted this silence to mean that the right to life of the unborn fetus takes priority over the right to life of the mother. Thus abused Catholic women make decisions alone, denied of the spiritual resources and support of a community that could help them in the midst of violent relationships (Nason-Clark et al. 2009).

Despite the androcentric bias of Catholic social teachings and their inadequate incorporation of a complex understanding of women's sexuality and violence, there are glimpses of a potential Canadian Catholic approach to problems of injustice that takes seriously women's reproductive choices. The social scientific study of religion and of Catholic social teachings as they pertain to women's sexuality and moral agency within a context of persistently high rates of domestic violence in Canada forms the background against which I now turn to a discussion of the voices of Catholic women.

Data and Methodology

I have collected qualitative data in several sociological studies of Catholics, including those who have joined the Catholic Network for Women's Equality (Holtmann 2008b), those who belong to women's religious orders, women in and out of the pews (Holtmann 2009, 2011), and those working in ministries related to the problem of domestic violence (Holtmann 2013). The data for three studies were collected in New Brunswick, and the data for a fourth study were collected in three dioceses in Atlantic, central, and western Canada. Although the latter included interviews with francophone Catholics, none of the research was conducted in the province of Quebec.[4] Data collection methods included focus groups and personal interviews with 123 people. Although the majority of research participants were women (N = 102), 20 of whom were nuns, men were also included (N = 21), 15 of whom were ordained. The analysis of the data reveals a rich complexity of ways that Catholic women grapple with issues related to religious and secular identities, gender, sexuality, personal agency, and action for social change. The variety of strategies that these Catholic women used when considering sexuality, religious agency, and social justice can be categorized in the following ways: (1) placing people before principles, (2) resisting a culture of silence, (3) fostering ministries of caring, and (4) building movements of religious change. Similar to the approach of Nason-Clark, Yip, and Boisvert in this volume, the strategies are explained here by referring to actual stories from the data.

Placing People before Principles

Julie[5] is a graduate student whose research focuses on women working in *maquiladora* factories in Mexico. In addition to attending mass regularly at a local parish, she is involved in a Catholic development and peace group on campus.[6] Julie spoke about the strong bond she had with her grandparents, who had played a significant role in her life after her mother divorced her abusive father. There was a time as a teenager when Julie stopped going to church. She describes herself as an agnostic during these years. As a doctoral student, she started going back to mass with some friends. Julie's first sexual experience was date rape. She did not tell anyone about this for years. Julie had also accompanied a friend to her abortion.

> I know what it was like to be raped. I was lucky enough not to be pregnant. I never had to make that decision. I can't ask another woman to carry the child of somebody that raped her. I don't feel it's my right to ask her to do that. I've read about the use of rape as a weapon of war ... So I can't tell these women that they don't have the right to an abortion, so I don't feel that I can say that I'm pro-life. I'm glad that abortion is legal because I don't want women to die ... doing it themselves, because in those extreme cases they're going to do it themselves ... But on the other hand, I will never be a militant for pro-choice, but I can't be a militant for pro-life either. So I'm somewhere in the middle ... Where's the right to life come in? So I'm obviously against capital punishment. I believe we don't have the right to take anyone's life. And abortion, I would say in the case of rape, I would approve. I would hope that the woman would choose to keep the child, but it's not my right to tell her what to do and to make her feel guilty for making that choice either.

Julie has a scholarly interest in women's issues and was engaged in both faith-based and secular forms of social action. She is familiar with the Catholic social teachings and believes in every person's right to life, yet she respects a woman's right to choose a safe abortion in cases of rape. Her story is typical of the kind of moral reasoning and agency used by Catholic women who participated in my research. She is reflexive about her Catholic identity in the light of women's experiences – both her own personal experience and the social scientific evidence. She is fully aware that violence against women is widespread. Her care for women and her consideration of difficulties posed by their circumstances are clear. She advocates respecting a woman's moral agency by giving her the right to decide what to do when she has been the victim of sexual violence and insists that she does not want to judge this decision, even though it is not the one that she would personally make because of her beliefs.

Julie's unwillingness to judge other women's choices and her awareness of the violent context in which women make these choices were echoed by many of the women who participated in my research, regardless of their age. For them, acting upon an awareness of the context in which women make moral decisions was a religious choice based on what they understood as the model of Jesus. Again and again, the women spoke of how they understood Jesus as someone who was accepting of others. He did not judge those who were on the margins of his society. For these Catholic women, Jesus's actions were about acceptance of and compassion for those adversely affected by structural injustice. Women who indicated that they publicly supported the church's right-to-life position were the minority in the sample. Among those who had taken a public pro-choice stance, concerns about late-term abortions informed a part of this choice.

The average age of the women in my research who were members of Catholic religious orders was sixty-five, with their time in religious orders averaging over forty years. They were very aware of the situations of female victims of violence and abuse in their local communities. As professionals in the fields of education, healthcare, therapeutic counselling, social work, and pastoral care, women religious had been in daily contact with women and children from a wide range of socio-economic backgrounds, especially the poor. Their communities were committed to serving the social needs of the marginalized in society. An example of this is Geraldine, a nun working as the volunteer co-ordinator of a local AIDS organization that offered assistance to the drug-addicted and to sex workers. The organization runs a needle exchange and a methadone clinic, and it distributes free contraception. She said that her work puts her "right where Jesus would be." She explained that her life had been a process of discovering more deeply what God was calling her to through the people she served. Geraldine spoke about her experiences as an elementary school teacher in an inner city:

> I know that a lot of those children were abused, and nobody ever told them that they loved them. It was a conversion moment for me too because I had just come from this crazy novitiate into God's love that accepts you unconditionally, and here I'm telling the children, and it's what's happening in me as well. That was a great learning process. And still in those times we were not allowed to touch the children, we were not to show any affection. But I couldn't help that because it was innate in me. So when I would bring them up to correct their work, I'd put my arm around them and we'd just correct the work together. I felt the touch for them was a healing, as [it was also] for me. It was natural. There wasn't anything that was off-colour or anything. It was just, "How many people have ever touched you today or yesterday?" I think I learned from the children's goodness, I learned about God from them. It was a real blessing.

The nuns shared stories about how working directly with the victims of violence and abuse had sensitized them to the circumstances of women and children in society. Ministry with survivors of abuse had an impact on their personal spiritualities and theological reflection. Geraldine refers to this as a "conversion" experience. The women religious spoke to me about how, through their professional work, they had become aware of their own victimization both within their orders and within the wider church structures.

In their compassionate consideration of the agency of women confronted with difficult reproductive choices in a context permeated by violence, the Catholic women in my research illustrate what Gilligan (2006, 204) refers to as a "moral perspective" of care. A care perspective places primacy on interdependent relationships in one's process of making moral choices. Gilligan contrasts this with a justice perspective that is focused on abstract principles of fairness – a perspective exemplified by most Catholic social teachings. According to Gilligan, women are more likely to take a care perspective in moral deliberations, perceiving an ethical problem within a context where relationships are central. This does not mean that by emphasizing caring, women are morally defective in comparison to men – they are different. Gilligan argues that a care perspective represents a way of knowing that complements the justice perspective. The two perspectives are valid alternatives in ethical deliberations, and used together they could create a needed sense of ambiguity in our construction and solution of moral problems (ibid., 204).[7] In placing embodied people before the principles of Catholic social teachings, Catholic women are exercising their religious agency through an ethic of caring. They are aware of the inadequacy of an exclusive justice perspective because of the reality of violence against women. A strict justice ethic, when it comes to reproductive choice, presumes that the context of the moral agent is violence-free and that moral agency is not compromised or affected by systemic factors. This is an incorrect assumption for the many women who experience sexual risk in their most intimate relationships (MacKinnon 2006). Given the reality of domestic violence, responsible for 52 percent of solved murders of women by their current or former intimate partners in Canada in 2008 (Johnson and Dawson 2010, 123), many Catholic women make reproductive choices that ensure life continues, while trying to respect the choices of others.

Resisting a Culture of Silence

The analysis of my data shows that Catholic women are frustrated with the culture of silence in most parishes regarding social issues, particularly as these relate to their families. In personal interviews and focus group discussions, many women spoke of how they wanted help discerning complicated moral issues but were dissatisfied with the leadership of priests. They were particularly critical of the ways that some priests preached about divorce.

Margot is a nurse who grew up in a strict Catholic family with ten siblings. She married young and her husband was violent. They separated when their second child was just three months old. For many years, she worked full time, raising her two children as a single parent without support from their father. She eventually remarried. During a focus group discussion, she spoke about her experience one Sunday:

> I was divorced and I sat in mass one time and my second husband was across the street at the United church, and I was sitting in the Catholic church while the priest gave a homily on divorce. And I looked around ... the church and I could see all these people that I knew that were divorced, all sitting there. "God, I can't believe he's saying this!" I was so mad ... And I came out and my husband was waiting for me, and I said, "I'm so mad, when I calm down I'm going back in to tell the priest just exactly

what he did." And he said, "Dear, what do you want to calm down for? Go back in now." I went back in and ... I was telling him what I thought of his sermon, and I said, "For once I want someone to take that same scripture and just talk about the pain that someone goes through when they experience a marriage breakdown" ... [He replied,] "Oh the next time it comes up ... I will preach differently." And I said, "Because if I hear a sermon like that again, I'm walking out." And do you know what? A couple years later the same thing came up. I'm in the middle of the church, he preached the same sermon, I picked up my coat and walked out – right down through the centre – can't not because I threatened I would. And I shook all the way down but I left. And really, it was demeaning and you know, the guilt, yes, it's exactly what I felt like too. That everything that goes wrong in your family then is because, you know, it's a divorce – *you* have had a divorce.

Margot's story is a vivid example of an attempt to convey the painful reality of a family breakup to a parish priest and one's church. She took a risk in speaking out and critiquing his homily. By walking out in the middle of mass during a subsequent homily on divorce, she held him accountable to his word.

Margot's actions were based on her experience of domestic violence and on moral standards of justice and care that were informed by her faith. Officially, Catholic women are not expected to remain in abusive relationships, and the church will annul marriages where violence and abuse have been a violation of the sacrament. Catholics seeking a marriage annulment must first be legally divorced. Priests who preach about divorce without acknowledging the reality of domestic violence are doing a grave disservice to their parishioners, at least one-third of whom have experienced some form of violence and long for a message of understanding from their religious leaders (Nason-Clark 1997, 41). Margot was clearly resisting the Catholic culture of silence when it came to violence, sexuality, and social justice.

Fostering Ministries of Caring

Many Catholic women are concerned about the future of their local churches. They spoke positively of the changes ushered in by the Second

Vatican Council – they were grateful that the fearful and coercive Catholicism of their youth had been replaced by one that embraced a God of love. They had taught this new theology to their children, few of whom have remained active Catholic adults. The women were insistent that their adult children were good people but knew that the Catholic faith was not central to their identities. One priest said that many Catholic families were like rubber bands – stretched to the point of breaking. Catholic women spoke about the pressures of contemporary life and how churches are not places where adult Catholics with careers and children can find understanding or support. Younger Catholics are turned away by what they perceive to be moralistic preaching. Women indicated that they wanted their churches to be communities of caring and compassion but added that they had often been frustrated in efforts to make this happen. Priests, parish councils, and certain individuals concerned with finances and adhering to narrow interpretations of the tradition were identified among the internal barriers to change. Too many churches were said to be emphasizing liturgical correctness at the expense of social action (Holtmann 2009). The evidence from my research suggests that women find it very difficult to foster ministries of caring at the parish level because of conflict and divisions. This is a problem given that the local parish is the central experience of religion for most Catholics (D'Antonio et al. 2001). Evidence of women's caring ministries can be found beyond the church walls.

Suzanne runs a shelter for trafficked women located in the downtown core of a Canadian city. She and her religious order have been involved in working against the trafficking of women in many countries throughout the world and as a nongovernmental organization at the United Nations. Suzanne felt a strong call from God to create a residential community for trafficked women. Suzanne knew that the city shelter accepted only women who had been abused by their husbands, but many migrant women were being victimized by brothers, uncles, grandfathers, or sponsors. She convinced a Catholic businessman and his Mennonite partner to purchase a large building and lease it at a reasonable cost to her religious order. The building includes a chapel, offices, and meeting spaces, as well as a residential facility with a kitchen and dorm-like bedrooms. Along with Isabel, another sister, Suzanne organizes everything at the shelter, including procuring priests to preside at daily masses in the chapel, networking with a variety of community agencies, educating church congregations about the problem of trafficking, and taking her turn cooking supper for the women with whom she lives. In its first five years, the shelter had been home to forty-one women from fifteen different countries with ten different religious backgrounds. Suzanne was convinced of the necessity of providing "a safe place where people are respected and loved and given chances and opportunities to grow." Suzanne spoke about the shelter's basis in faith and about the contradictions within the Catholic Church:

> The purpose here is to create a home. I don't pretend that I'm going to help teach them all English and get them jobs and solve their traumas. But all of that happens – all of it happens. I think, you know, for me the basic premise is the incarnation. I mean, that's the word is made flesh and made flesh in all people. And when it comes to women, they are the most disenfranchised people in the world – women and children. And the whole thing with patriarchy drives me absolutely wild. And that's an issue within the church that is very hard to claim. Well, I think it is in the world, but it's very hard to claim. People don't see themselves that way – don't see themselves as abusing women by not allowing them on an equal playing field in terms of decision making or whatever. So that's an ongoing struggle and I take it on when I can.

In taking on the struggle against patriarchy and abuse, Suzanne had to defend the shelter's work to the bishop, who was upset that she was recruiting retired priests in the diocese to celebrate daily mass. She said that the bishop was probably initially threatened by her work because he did not understand it. With time, he became very supportive. Suzanne's faith and persistence in caring for abused immigrant women in the face of resistance from the bishop paid off. She said, "I'm so proud to be Catholic, like I mean that's the truth, for all of the rottenness, the brokenness … the truth is that I am the church and [Isabel] is and you are and so that's the church. It's not just the hierarchy and it is the hierarchy because some of them are really good."

Building Movements for Religious Change

Because it is very difficult to develop ministries of caring in parishes or to have public discussions about Catholic social teachings and issues of concern to women, some Catholic women have formed movements for religious change. This can be understood as a contemporary rendering of the tradition of establishing Catholic religious communities (Holtmann 2008a). Women's religious and moral agency has become a matter of social justice. It has become fundamentally problematic for Catholic women to engage collectively in social justice work when the institution remains a place of structural injustice, particularly in regards to issues of gender and sexuality. Women are working to create explicitly Catholic spaces where their feminist religious identities are affirmed (Howard Ecklund 2005) and where their agency in the work for social justice can flourish and be celebrated rather than held suspect.

Martha is a social worker who enjoys gardening with her husband. They had immigrated to Canada from the United States years ago. Before marrying, Martha had participated in student demonstrations against the Vietnam War. She said, "I felt very strongly that we shouldn't be in the war. I had six brothers – half of whom were eligible for the draft." Martha said that she valued nonviolence and that when the student marches turned to riots, she got really scared. She remembered the shooting of four students at Kent State and said that she still did not feel comfortable in crowds. Settling into a new community in Canada, Martha had helped to form a woman's consciousness-raising group with other young mothers. "We'd meet at different people's houses and talk about issues concerning women ... That was when the book *Our Bodies, Our Selves*, that was when that came out. That was like a bible ... We talked about health issues and parenting – a lot of parenting." Martha is a lector in her parish, and since she is a social worker, her life is about doing good works. But she longed for a deeper spiritual basis for her work. She had tried to form a social justice group but without success. Her frustration was palpable:

> It's not a healthy church – it's very unhealthy and I don't care what people say about the church – it's made up of humans. I think it's a very sick organization – really, really. I could go on ... but how could they have all that money when people are starving and dying of AIDS? How do you read the gospel and sit in Vatican City and wear all those robes? I flat out don't know – it just takes my breath away. How can you do that? How can you? It's a mystery to me ... It drives me crazy, but I still go to church, because I believe that we need to be together. I think we need a

community – it's the community I grew up with. There's so many good individuals in the church ... I can accept humanness on the individual level, but on the institutional level of the church ... That's what sent me away in the '70s – I couldn't stand going to church while the Vietnam War was going on and people never even mentioned it ... and even now ... if [the priests are] supposed to be helping us connect, how can you do that and not talk about Canada in Afghanistan? How can you not address that? How does that not be a spiritual issue? It's a mystery to me. I need help with this stuff! I may be fifty-eight, almost fifty-nine, but I still need help trying to sort this stuff out. To me, the church does very little to help. They only talk about the individual, like, "Be good to your neighbour." But my neighbour is in Afghanistan and in Africa.

Martha had joined a local chapter of the Catholic Network for Women's Equality. She found a religious context where she could voice her frustrations, ask tough questions, and continue to develop an adult faith life. She is an educated professional who understands the connections between the social problems in her local community – poverty, substance abuse, sexuality – and the global problems of war and the AIDS pandemic. She is trying to make a difference yet is longing for the spiritual wisdom of her Catholic heritage and the support of a spiritual community. Her frustration with her parish led her to seek out a space where she could also consider social issues with other women by drawing on a creative mix of Catholic social teachings, feminist theology, scripture, economics, and politics.

Conclusions

The stories of Julie, Margot, Suzanne, Isabel, and Martha show that the Catholic women in my research utilized the resources of their faith in imaginative ways to deal with the paradoxes of their church. This was particularly true when it came to issues of sexuality and reproductive choice in contexts of high rates of domestic violence in Canada. In placing themselves and the flesh and blood people whom they knew and loved before the abstract principles of Catholic social teaching, particularly as they pertain to reproductive choice, these women made moral decisions based on a relational ethic of caring. The lived reality of actual relationships with boyfriends, husbands, children, friends, and persons living in poverty superseded the abstract principles proclaimed by distant bishops or popes. These women resisted the Catholic hierarchy's silence concerning domestic violence and trafficking in part by creating cultures of caring that were inspired by the example of Jesus. This is not easy to do given that the rhetoric of religious leaders does not affirm such efforts. Some women are finding ways to move beyond the inertia of their local parishes. On the basis of their own experiences of exclusion, religious and/ or secular, they have reached out to the marginalized in their midst: the victims of rape, women who decide to get an abortion, those who have experienced the pain of divorce, children and youth who have been neglected or abused, families struggling with the conditions imposed by a neoliberal economic system that values profits over people, and Catholic women who desire religious leadership.

More often than not, the culture of caring that Catholic women create does not take place immediately within their local churches. For many, it is evidenced in the nonviolent and egalitarian family relationships they share with their children and grandchildren. Vowed religious communities are traditional Catholic spaces somewhere between the hierarchy and the people in the pews where imaginative reinterpretations of scripture and tradition serve a social action agenda. Women in these spaces utilize their declining material resources and abundant religious hope to serve the oppressed. Sometimes resistance takes the form of alternative organizations or small groups, somewhat like the space that religious communities offer but frequently without the sanction of Catholic clergy. These alternative organizations and groups usually operate in parallel with the church, enabling women to maintain some form of connection to larger Catholic structures. In these spaces, women are supported in their attempts to perceive, conceive, and live with the tensions created by the paradoxes in the contemporary Canadian Catholic Church.

Notes

1 Similarly, Trothen's (Chapter 8, this volume) analysis of elite level sport highlights how the agency of athletes is situated within the discourse of sport, which simultaneously promotes "natural" athletic achievement and unbridled techno-science in the pursuit of profit. Trothen posits that a theological justice ethic demands that those

involved in sport – athletes, promoters, governments, and fans – consider the larger implications of such a system, particularly for people who fall outside the socially constructed boundaries of "normal."

2 There is considerable resistance to sexual dimorphism within Catholic theological circles and among Catholics. Nearly every person in my research disagreed with the church's condemnation of homosexuality and same-sex marriage.

3 Pope Benedict XVI has stated that for some individuals – for instance, a male prostitute – the use of a condom to prevent HIV infection may be a first step toward assuming moral responsibility (Pope Benedict XVI and Seewald 2010, 119). It is unclear at this stage whether this can be applied to situations concerning women's sexuality, particularly when a woman considers her life to be in danger.

4 Francophone Catholics differ substantially from their anglophone counterparts on issues of ecclesial authority, personal autonomy, and sexuality (Couture 2008).

5 This is a pseudonym, as are all the other names used for research participants in this chapter.

6 This group is the Canadian Catholic Organization for Development and Peace, an international nongovernmental organization founded by the Canadian bishops over forty years ago to raise awareness and mobilize Catholics in support of the struggles of the global poor.

7 Gilligan's (2006, 204) case for women's use of a "moral perspective" of care is problematic for some feminists because of its essentialism. MacKinnon (2006) argues that women's sexuality is socially constructed as different from men's by patriarchy and that an affirmation of difference is an affirmation of patriarchy. Catholic women who choose to engage in social justice work within the church must address the patriarchal structures that they wish to reform, and these structures include moral principles.

References

Ammerman, N.T. 2003. Religious Identities and Religious Institutions. In *Handbook of the Sociology of Religion,* ed. M. Dillon, 207-24. Cambridge: Cambridge University Press.

Archer, M.S. 2007. *Making Our Way through the World: Human Reflexivity and Social Mobility.* Cambridge: Cambridge University Press.

Baggett, J. 2009. *Sense of the Faithful: How American Catholics Live Their Faith.* New York: Oxford University Press.

Beattie, T. 2010. Dialogue, Difference and Human Development: Gendered Perspectives on Catholic Social Teaching. Lecture presented at St. Thomas University, Fredericton, New Brunswick, 11 February. https://sites.google.com/site/tinabeattie/papers.

Bouclin, M.E. 2006. *Seeking Wholeness: Women Dealing with Abuse of Power in the Catholic Church.* Collegeville, MN: Liturgical Press.

Canadian Conference of Catholic Bishops. 2000. To Live without Fear. *With Respect to Women: A History of CCCB Initiatives Concerning Women in the Church and Society, 1971-2000,* 73-77. Ottawa: Concacan.

Canadian Press. 2010. Archbishop Defends Abortion Comments; Roman Catholic Primate of Canada Said Abortion Is Unjustifiable, Even for Rape. *Moncton Times and Transcript,* 27 May.

Catholics for Choice. 2014. *The Facts Tell the Story: Catholics and Choice.* http://www.catholicsforchoice.org/topics/catholicsandchoice/documents/Factstellthestoryweb.pdf.

COLF (Catholic Organization for Life and Family). 2013. Publications on "Family Topics." http://www.colf.ca/index.php/en/publications/family-issues.

Congregation for the Doctrine of the Faith. 2012. *Doctrinal Assessment of the Leadership Conference of Women Religious.* http://www.usccb.org/about/doctrine/doctrinal-assessment-for-lcwr.cfm.

Couture, D. 2008. Feminist Theologies in Quebec: Interspirituality of the Feminine Divine. In *Feminist Theology with a Canadian Accent: Canadian Perspectives on Contextual Feminist Theology,* ed. M.A. Beavis, E. Guillemin, and B. Pell, 58-77. Toronto: Novalis.

D'Antonio, W.V., J.D. Davidson, D.R. Hoge, and K. Meyer. 2001. *American Catholics: Gender, Generation, and Commitment.* Walnut Creek, CA: Altamira.

D'Antonio, W.V., and A. Pogorelc. 2007. *Voices of the Faithful: Loyal Catholics Striving for Change.* New York: Crossroads.

Dillon, M. 1999. *Catholic Identity: Balancing Reason, Faith and Power.* Cambridge: Cambridge University Press.

Dunne, V. 2008. A Force of Nature: Canadian Catholic Women Shifting the Ecclesial Landscape. In *Feminist Theology with a Canadian Accent: Canadian Perspectives on Contextual Feminist Theology,* ed. M.A. Beavis, E. Guillemin, and B. Pell, 179-99. Toronto: Novalis.

Ebaugh, H.R. 1993. *Women in the Vanishing Cloister: Organizational Decline in Catholic Religious Orders in the United States.* New Brunswick, NJ: Rutgers University Press.

Flannery, A., ed. 1988. *Vatican Council II: The Conciliar and Post-conciliar Documents.* Rev. ed. Northport, NY: Costello.

Gervais, C.L.M. 2012. Canadian Women Religious' Negotiation of Feminism and Catholicism. *Sociology of Religion* 73 (4): 384-410.

Gilligan, C. 2006. Moral Orientation and Moral Development. In *Theorizing Feminisms: A Reader,* ed. E. Hackett and S. Haslanger, 200-10. New York: Oxford University Press.

Gunn, J., and M. Lambton. 1999. *Calling Out the Prophetic Tradition: A Jubilee of Social Teaching from the Canadian Conference of Catholic Bishops.* Ottawa: CCCB Publications.

Hartsock, N. 1998. *The Feminist Standpoint Revisited and Other Essays*. Boulder, CO: Westview.

Holtmann, C. 2008a. My Sister My Self: Women Religious at Work. Paper presented at the annual meeting of the Society for the Sociology of Religion, Boston, Massachusetts, 31 July.

–. 2008b. Resistance Is Beautiful: The Growth of the Catholic Network for Women's Equality in New Brunswick. In *Feminist Theology with a Canadian Accent: Canadian Perspectives on Contextual Feminist Theology*, ed. M.A. Beavis, E. Guillemin, and B. Pell, 200-19. Toronto: Novalis.

–. 2009. Heart, Mind and Soul: Catholic Women and Social Action. MA thesis, University of New Brunswick.

–. 2011. Workers in the Vineyard: Catholic Women and Social Action. In *Religion, Spirituality and Everyday Practice*, ed. W. Swatos and G. Giordan, 141-52. New York: Springer.

–. 2013. From the Top: What Does It Mean When Catholic Bishops Speak Out on Issues of Family Violence? *Strengthening Families and Ending Abuse: Churches and Their Leaders Look to the Future*, ed. N. Nason-Clark, B. Fisher-Townsend, and V. Fahlberg, 139-59. Eugene, OR: Wipf and Stock.

Howard Ecklund, E. 2005. Different Identity Accounts for Catholic Women. *Review of Religious Research* 47 (2): 135-49.

–. 2006. Organizational Culture and Women's Leadership: A Study of Six Parishes. *Sociology of Religion* 67 (1): 81-98.

Hunt, M.E. 2005. Just Good Sex: Feminist Catholicism and Human Rights. In *Good Sex: Feminist Perspectives from the World's Religions*, ed. P. Beattie Jung, M.E. Hunt, and R. Balakrishnan, 158-73. New Brunswick, NJ: Rutgers University Press.

Johnson, H., and M. Dawson. 2010. *Violence against Women in Canada: Research and Policy Perspectives*. New York: Oxford University Press.

Korteweg, A.C. 2008. The Sharia Debate in Ontario: Gender, Islam and Representations of Muslim Women's Agency. *Gender and Society* 22 (4): 434-54.

MacKinnon, C. 2006. Desire and Power. In *Theorizing Feminisms: A Reader*, ed. E. Hackett and S. Haslanger, 256-65. New York: Oxford University Press.

Maguire, D.C. 1984. *Reflections of a Catholic Theologian on Visiting an Abortion Clinic*. https://www.catholicsforchoice.org/topics/reform/documents/2000reflectionsofacatholictheologian.pdf.

Mahmood, S. 2001. Feminist Theory, Embodiment, and the Docile Agent: Some Reflections on the Egyptian Islamic Revival. *Cultural Anthropology* 16 (2): 202-36.

McGuire, M.B. 2008. *Lived Religion: Faith and Practice in Everyday Life*. New York: Oxford University Press.

Nason-Clark, N. 1997. *The Battered Wife: How Christian Families Confront Family Violence*. Louisville, KY: Westminster John Knox Press.

Nason-Clark, N., and B. Fisher-Townsend. 2005. Gender. In *Handbook of Religion and Social Institutions,* ed. H.R. Ebaugh, 207-23. New York: Springer.

Nason-Clark, N., C. Holtmann, B. Fisher-Townsend, S. McMullin, and L. Ruff. 2009. The RAVE Project: Developing Web-Based Religious Resources for Social Action on Domestic Violence. *Critical Social Work* 10 (1). http://www1.uwindsor.ca/criticalsocialwork/the-rave-project-developing-web-based-religious-resources-for-social-action-on-domestic-abuse.

Pew Research Center. 2008. *U.S. Religious Landscape Survey – Religious Affiliation: Diverse and Dynamic.* http://religions.pewforum.org/pdf/report-religious-landscape-study-full.pdf.

Pfeil, M.R. 2008. Wise as Serpents, Innocent as Doves: Strategic Appropriation of Catholic Social Teaching. In *Prophetic Witness: Catholic Women's Strategies for Reform,* ed. C.M. Griffith, 64-71. New York: Herder and Herder.

Pontifical Council for Justice and Peace. 2005. *Compendium of the Social Doctrine of the Church.* Ottawa: CCCB Publications.

Pope Benedict XVI. 2009. *Caritas in Veritate.* http://www.vatican.va/holy_father/benedict_xvi/encyclicals/documents/hf_ben-xvi_enc_20090629_caritas-in-veritate_en.html.

Pope Benedict XVI, and Peter Seewald. 2010. *Light of the World: The Pope, the Church and the Signs of the Times.* Trans. M.J. Miller and A.J. Walker. San Francisco: Ignatius.

Pope John Paul II. 1995. *Evangelium Vitae.* http://www.vatican.va/holy_father/john_paul_ii/encyclicals/documents/hf_jp-ii_enc_25031995_evangelium-vitae_en.html.

Radford Ruether, R. 1986. *Women-Church: Theology and Practice of Feminist Liturgical Communities.* San Francisco: Harper and Row.

–. 2006. Women, Reproductive Rights and the Catholic Church. May. https://www.catholicsforchoice.org/topics/reform/documents/2006womenreproductiverightsandthecatholicchurch.asp.

Social Affairs Commission of the Assembly of Quebec Bishops. 1989. *A Heritage of Violence: A Pastoral Reflection on Conjugal Violence.* Montreal: Social Affairs Committee of the Assembly of Quebec Bishops.

Squires, N. 2013. Pope Francis Hails Women as Book Reveals Teenage Infatuation. *Telegraph* (London), 3 April. http://www.telegraph.co.uk/news/religion/the-pope/9969334/Pope-Francis-hails-women-as-book-reveals-teenage-infatuation.html.

Ternier-Gommers, M. 2007. *Catholic Women in Ministry: Changing the Way Things Are.* Ottawa: Novalis.

United Nations. 2008. *UNite to End Violence against Women: UN Secretary-General's Campaign.* http://www.un.org/en/women/endviolence/pdf/VAW.pdf.

–. 2010. *We Can End Poverty: Millennium Development Goals and Beyond 2015.* http://www.un.org/millenniumgoals.

Van Pelt Campbell, G. 2007. Religion and Phases of Globalization. In *Religion, Globalization and Culture,* ed. P. Beyer and L. Beamann, 281-302. Boston: Brill.

Wallace, R. 1992. *They Call Her Pastor: A New Role for Catholic Women.* Albany, NY: SUNY Press.

Wilde, M. 2007. *Vatican II: A Sociological Analysis of Religious Change.* Princeton, NJ: Princeton University Press.

Winter, M.T., A. Lumis, and A. Stokes. 1995. *Defecting in Place: Women Claiming Responsibility for Their Own Spiritual Lives.* New York: Crossroads.

Wittberg, P. 1994. *The Rise and Fall of Catholic Religious Orders: A Social Movement Perspective.* Albany, NY: SUNY Press.

–. 2006. *From Piety to Professionalism – and Back? Transformations of Organized Religious Virtuosity.* New York: Lexington Books.

World March of Women. 2000. *Advocacy Guide to Women's World Demands: Eliminating Poverty.* http://www.worldmarchofwomen.org/publications/cahier/c_03/en/base_view.

PART 3
Sexual Bodies/Religious Bodies

THIS LAST SECTION is comprised of chapters that consider different moments of the embodied character of sexualities and religions. Any conception of fixed, static boundaries separating religious and sexual embodied identities is firmly challenged by these remaining chapters; each highlights the permeable lines between religious, sexual, political, and social spheres.

The authors in this section point to the compromised but often persistent and creative exercise of agency by those who experience abusive, coercive, or at least limiting environments. Coping strategies, including those observed by Andrew Kam-Tuck Yip and Catherine Holtmann in the previous section, are portrayed vividly in the embodied examples provided by saints, sport, and domestic violence. The subversive and transformative potential of both religious and sexual subjects is a repeated theme.

While acknowledging the limited truth held in any one fluid narrative moment, all three authors use narratives to illuminate arguments or claims. Resources for reimaging the many intersections of sexuality and religion in constraining or punishing contexts are identified in these chapters. It is curious that often those who are defined as exceptional in either a heroic or severely marginalized manner hold power to destabilize normative constructions. These chapters illuminate the power of particular subjects to resist normative frameworks and reductionist rhetoric.

This section can inspire readers to think more critically about the many and varied locations of sexual and religious diversity. Further, these chapters will assist readers in exploring the meaning of these identities, as the chapters provide some far-reaching and perhaps surprising points of intersection.

In Chapter 7, consistent with feminist theories, Donald Boisvert draws on segments of his own life narrative to illuminate Roman Catholic teachings about sexuality through the use of young saints as role models. He argues that official Roman Catholicism uses these saints to uphold sexual norms and values that stifle sexual and religious diversity. Through narrative and the application of theory, Boisvert suggests that stories of saints can have surprisingly ambiguous effects on identity formation.

Using two examples of young saints – Maria Goretti and Dominic Savio – Boisvert suggests that normative male sexual desire is projected onto these idealized and constructed narratives of saints. Goretti died protecting her virginity, and for this she was canonized and looked to as a model of virtue and purity for girls and young women. Savio felt called to become a priest as a young child. Accordingly, he lived his young life with emphasis on obedience, piety, and chastity, being careful always to conceal his body. Boisvert points out the ambiguities of Savio's story, noting hints at same-sex attraction and his "effeminate" disposition.

Subversively, Boisvert proposes alternative ways of hearing these saints by considering them as agents. To do this, Boisvert recounts some of his own story. Instead of gender-specific shaming messages about the pre-eminence of bodily purity and chastity for girls (even over life itself) and about abstinence from "self-abuse" (masturbation) for boys, a young Boisvert saw the liberating ambiguous and attractive sexual promise in these saints. Through this unintended perception, Boisvert's Catholic upbringing gave him the resources to claim and celebrate his own sexual particularity and desires, subverting the "official Catholic narrative" (akin to Yip's findings). He explains, "I was also a young boy struggling with an emerging sense of sexual difference. Saints' stories normalized this difference. Their queer, non-normative lives mirrored and revalued my own." Boisvert shows that how these stories are told is shaped by the narrator's perspective and power. His bottom line is that subversive readings cannot be shut out: "Saints don't always do what the church tells them to do."

In Chapter 8, Tracy Trothen explores the complex intersection of technoscience, sport, and religion, asking what the implications of this intersection are for embodiment and sexualities. For some, Trothen points out, sport serves as an alternative way of being religious. Sport, as a secular religion, is not only an example of the increasing religious diversity in North American society but also transgressively claims the body as a spiritual locus; Trothen suggests that sport as a secular religion challenges the normative sacred-profane bifurcation that devalues the body.

Innovations in sport enhancement are making existing embodiment diversity more visible and are adding to this diversity. For example, science offers medical tests to reveal hormone levels and other so-called determinants of sex. Genetic modification technologies may make it possible in the future for athletes to increase their endurance capacities. And prosthetic limb technologies are allowing athletes without legs such as Oscar Pistorius to compete in the Olympics. Whether these embodiment differences are fair in athletic competition has been the subject of much debate. Using the narrative examples of elite athletes Oscar Pistorius and Caster Semenya, Trothen challenges the ways that the enhancement debate is being framed, pointing to the implications for religious and sexual diversity. She argues that if embodiment diversity – and, with it, sexual diversity – is to be seen and valued, the underlying assumptions that frame contemporary approaches to the sport enhancement debate, including essentialist understandings of gender and sex, must be identified and challenged.

Trothen shows that the merging of sport as a religion with techno-science destabilizes preconceived embodiment categories, including ways of being sexual. This destabilizaton, she proposes, creates potential for the retrenchment of exclusionary religious and sexual norms as well as potential for increased awareness and inclusion of diverse and fluid sexual-religious identities. Similar to Nancy Nason-Clark, she sees embodiment as necessarily concerning sexuality and explores this connection throughout the chapter.

In Chapter 9, Nancy Nason-Clark investigates the relationship of women's experiences of domestic violence to their religious and sexual identities. Nason-Clark underscores the resourcefulness of these women in working out their identities both as women with abused bodies and as women of faith and strong spirits. These stories of abuse and survival include themes of agency re/claimed and creative imaginings of just relationships. Methodologically, she draws on quantitative and qualitative research mostly on conservative Protestant Canadian women. Similar to Boisvert, Trothen, and others in this volume, she uses narrative to illustrate and enliven her arguments.

Nason-Clark critiques normative, conservative Christian ideals about sexual purity, contending that these values leave women even more open to deep damage from abuse, particularly when they are unable to protect themselves sexually. Women who are committed Christians are even more vulnerable to abuse because of persistent conservative theological convictions that perpetuate abuse. The power of such erroneous and damaging "religious rhetoric" is illustrated by several authors in this volume.

Nason-Clark identifies what is perhaps an even more powerful factor than these theological convictions: fear. She contends that fear can stop women from leaving or getting help, that fear of not being competent to handle disclosures of abuse due to inadequate seminary education can prevent pastors from speaking out about abuse or from making referrals, and that fear fosters mutual suspicion between social agencies and faith communities. In short, fear threatens to protect abusers. Nason-Clark concludes that amazingly, even in the face of fear, women often reclaim their agency, making stubborn inroads toward inclusivity and justice through their faith, communal strength, and resilience.

– Tracy J. Trothen

7

The Construction of a Sexual Pedagogy
CHILDHOOD AND SAINTS IN ROMAN CATHOLIC DISCOURSE

Donald L. Boisvert

There is a photo from when my brother and I were children that shows us kneeling in front of a statue of Our Lady of Fatima in our home. I was probably six or so, and my brother may have been five. We are in our pyjamas. I am kneeling very erect, with my hands clasped, staring intently at the Virgin. My brother is sitting on the floor, not very religious at all, looking rather sadly at the camera. Quite apart from what this says about our respective personalities, I am struck by my posture and my apparent look of pious intensity. It's obvious that here was a young Catholic body very well aligned with the dictates of his church and displaying the proper devotional attitude and reverence. Here was a young Catholic body moulded by the discipline of Catholicism.

I want to write about young Catholic bodies, both of this world and not, both my own and those of others. In Christianity, as well as in broader Western culture, the liminal bodies of the young have always been seen as suspicious entities. They are perceived as unfinished and anarchistic, needing the hands of experienced adults to mould them. They require discipline and the imposition of limits and constraints. These are unruly bodies, made particularly risky and dangerous by an emerging – and often confused and confusing – sexuality. Yet a great deal of cultural taboo surrounds this sexuality of the young. We would rather not imagine or think of the bodies of the young as being sexual (in fact, we are not allowed to do so), even though the media are constantly projecting nubile, semi-naked images meant to serve ever-expanding market needs. In religious worlds, the bodies of the young are more often than not bearers of hazard, for the bodies of the young remain incomplete, murky, unsettled. Their innocence implies lack; their emptiness needs to be filled by other sorts of wild imaginings. In Catholic culture, evil always hovers around innocence (Orsi 2005, 78-89).

In most patriarchal religion, nonmale, nonadult, and nonheterosexual bodies are viewed not only with a measure of suspicion but also with a certain amount of fear, respect, and awe. These "unbounded" bodies of women, of children, and of those considered sexually marginal can, in fact, be framed and treated as uniquely powerful sources of spiritual enlightenment. Their seemingly bottomless physicality and their non-normative quality act as ciphers onto which can be projected the desires, needs, and fantasies of male authority. Bodies that are located on the margins of – and that are made subservient to – male normativity are always expected to undergird orthodox desire, whether sexual or religious. Such bodies are constructs and projections of normative male need and of church-infused discourse and imagery. In a Roman Catholic Church that remains dominated by male clerical authority, this question assumes a particular relevance and urgency – for it cannot be simply coincidental that youth, most often known and revered for their innocence and bodily purity, occupy such a privileged position in the pantheon of Catholic holy persons. How do such holy youth, in fact, serve as projections of, or foils for, masculine clerical desire?

Orsi (2005, 74) speaks of the "corporalization of the sacred," which implies "the practice of rendering the invisible visible by constituting it as an experience in a body – in one's own body or in someone else's body – so that the experiencing body itself becomes the bearer of presence for oneself and for others." Ambivalence characterizes young bodies in religious contexts, thereby requiring that they be framed in adult terms. "Children's bodies, rationalities, imaginations, and desires have all been privileged media for giving substance to religious meaning, for making the sacred present and material, not only *for* children but *through* them too, for adults in relation to them" (ibid., 77, emphasis in original). Written or carved onto the bodies of the young, the holy emerges as a meeting place for adult needs and desires, for their embodiment in the raw and imperfect materiality of children and youth.

North American Catholic culture developed a wide array of strategies – most often overseen and administered by nuns and teaching brothers – to tame and control the bodies of Catholic youth. This chapter examines the church's use of adolescent Catholic saints to construct and appropriate a sort of Catholic sexual pedagogy for youth. My timeframe is the first six to seven decades of the twentieth century in North America, until about the end of the 1960s. This era also saw the emergence of adolescence as a distinctive life stage and the development of a unique teenage culture very often fuelled by unfolding consumer needs. My broader intent, within the context of the larger diversity project that has inspired this volume, is to examine some of the ways that religion, as a cultural system, inculcates the young with sexual norms and values that can often inhibit or negate an inclusive understanding of both sexual and religious diversity.

Catholic boys were always being encouraged to be vigilant about their bodies, to respect them as "dwelling places of the Holy Spirit." Sex was not talked about directly in Catholic school, although we were clearly all aware that we should not "touch ourselves" improperly. This was spoken in veiled ways, the admission of guilt being quantitatively rattled off in the darkness of the confessional box: "Bless me, Father, for I have committed the sin of self-abuse six times in the past week ..." Here is yet another example of silence speaking louder than words. Through the technical language of "self-abuse," we were declaring ourselves incapable of sexual discipline and therefore susceptible to all sorts of spiritually dangerous forms of sexual difference.

Notes on Methodology

This chapter presents a discussion of how religious identity can be embodied. In doing so, it uses imagination and narrative as key methodological tools. Several italicized anecdotes and reflections (snapshots, if you will) from my own life as a Catholic youth are interspersed between more properly "academic" sections that provide a general analysis of the phenomenon of the young Catholic saint. A threefold purpose guides this approach. First, in line with feminist scholarship, I believe strongly in the importance of using one's personal experience as a source of scholarly reflection and analysis, particularly when it comes to questions of gender, sexuality, and the body. Second, my approach is meant to ground my analysis in direct and tangible contexts by using existential insight as both a marker and a reflection of identity. Third, I hope to provide the reader with a more engaging and insightful account. Fellow authors in this volume (Nancy Nason-Clark, Heather Shipley, Tracy Trothen, and Andrew Kam-Tuck Yip) likewise address various aspects of the intersections between narrative and identity construction.

Stories – one's own or those of others – provide an especially powerful and dynamic lens through which religious experience can be read and appropriated. In her introduction to *Martyrdom and Memory,* Elizabeth A. Castelli (2004) recalls the time when she and her young Catholic schoolmates had to choose a specific saint's name for the sacrament of confirmation they were about to receive. Not only were there gendered differences in how the girls and the boys went through the selection process (the boys being far more carefree about the whole thing), but the names chosen by the girls were also clearly intended to imbue them with a different sort of identity. As Castelli (ibid., 3) explains,

> After all, the selection of one's saint was not a matter of locating someone whose story was decidedly similar to one's own. The saints' lives were not *our* lives; indeed, their *differences* were precisely the point. The chance to choose one's own name was rather an opportunity to embrace a new story, one that appeared in higher contrast and brighter intensity in the illustrations of the books where hagiographies were found. *Their* lives were *not* ours, but we could bask in their reflected glory by taking their names and copying out their stories into our notebooks. (Emphasis in original)

Like stories of martyrdom in early Christian communities, Castelli (ibid., 4) calls this "a form of culture making, whereby Christian identity was indelibly marked by the collective memory of the religious suffering of others." Castelli and her friends were engaging in memory work, a process that, although it may have endowed them with a new and different identity, more importantly linked them to a whole narrative of heroic Christian witness. This helped them to cement a sense of an ongoing and atemporal Catholic community. It is this work of memory – the merging of one's identity with that of a broader community of Christian (or Catholic) heroic witness – that also motivated me in my own youthful identification with adolescent saints. This identification not only helped me to make sense of my own emerging desires, both religious and sexual, but also linked me to an entire host of heroic and inspiring heavenly companions with whom I could converse in my intimate and solitary moments as a teenager. And they were so different from me, so much more saintly and heroic than I was!

It is not my intent that my experience be seen as paradigmatic or representative; rather, its similarity to others' experiences is a question of degrees but also of constructing and demonstrating a sense of continuity. I was a young Catholic boy. I was educated in the ways of Catholic culture. My young Catholic body was signified through Catholic values and imagery, and mine was a body imprinted with the markings and reflected desires of a certain Catholic sexual pedagogy. I developed close affinities with young Catholic saints. But I was not unique in this regard. Scores of other young Catholic boys, from different generations, would have experienced something similar. But I cannot speak of or for these others because I am not them. I can, however, speak with my own voice in the hope that others can mark their experience in continuity with mine. This is the work of memory, where we forge identity and build meaning from a similar pool of experience. Essentially, I am constructing a Catholic body in these pages, and my stories are instances of how a Catholic body was, in fact, put together. Others may want to reflect on how their young Catholic bodies fitted with mine. If they find echoes, we have constructed memory together.

The question can and has been asked: what does it mean, from a scholarly perspective, to construct memory together? Specifically, I can ask: what differentiates my constructed Catholic memory of saints – or of the meanings attached to my Catholic upbringing – from other sorts of memories, some considerably less pious or even illegitimate? In a way, this question can be seen as misleading, for it suggests that a feminist or queer reading of one's experience does not constitute a legitimate source of, or venue for, serious scholarly reflection. I reject such a presupposition. It denigrates and minimizes the full panoply of human experience – especially that of marginality – as invalid and unworthy of serious intellectual analysis. Nonetheless, as I mentioned earlier, I do not wish to suggest that my experience of Roman Catholicism was and is normative or that there is a sort of monolithic Catholic Church exclusively reflective of this experience. There is not, nor has there ever been. What makes my analysis a scholarly reading, therefore, is the way that, with the help of the work of other scholars, I critically analyze categories of the body, youth, and sanctity. I try to build connections where none may appear at first glance. In a way, one could say that scholarship is art. Of course, my experience is important and relevant, which is why I use it. But it is not normative in any absolute way, which is why I italicize it. But it certainly is legitimate and proper.

Bodies and sexuality are notoriously slippery, even more so when religion is added into the mix. So, too, is desire, for the lines between religious and sexual desire are often porous in the extreme. Religion stands as an eminently queer thing, the place of all possibilities: the site of imagination, open bodies, fluid identities, and ever shifting visions of the self and of others. Narrative helps to keep open these possibilities, for it displays and constructs memory. I suggest that Catholicism is framed by a narrative of desire. It taught me and countless others how to be not only sexual but also most definitely and defiantly queer in both our sexual and our religious yearnings and choices. Catholicism also forecloses a great deal that is sexual. Consequently, it binds rather than opens up, limits rather than uncovers, seals rather than unlocks. Thus there is a great deal of ambivalence in the Catholic worldview. It has often imposed a closed paradigm, one that resists openness to diversity and difference, particularly of a sexual nature. Grounded in a specifically Roman Catholic perspective, my intent, more broadly, remains to understand what it is about sexuality that so distresses some religious traditions and thereby to obtain a sharper and more nuanced sense of how these traditions may go about projecting this angst onto, and actualizing this angst within, their adherents. Devotion to young saints is one such strategy of projection and embodiment.

I remember when it came time for me to make my confirmation. I was actually in fifth grade at the time. But since I had gone from an American to a Canadian school, I was following confirmation classes with the children in first grade. It felt quite awkward. I was told I had to pick a confirmation name, something that would mark me off as a mature Catholic believer. We were instructed that it had to be an easy name, but more important, that of a saint. I was at a bit of a loss, until I remembered the name of my best friend: Christopher. I picked that as my confirmation name. This was, of course, before St. Christopher was demoted from the saintly pantheon. I'm pretty sure I had a crush on my friend Christopher. No doubt my choice of name was meant as a token of my affection for him. I remember I was genuinely excited about telling him but was disappointed by his reaction. He seemed rather indifferent. My first broken heart.

Saint Making as Pedagogical Work

It is a well-known fact that John Paul II beatified and canonized more individuals than all of his papal predecessors combined, exactly 1,820 in total. He himself was declared blessed by his successor, Benedict XVI, on 1 May 2011, and declared a saint by Pope Francis in 2014. Saint making has always been regarded in the Roman Catholic Church as pedagogical work of the highest order, and John Paul II understood this better than any other pope in history. He saw the making of saints – saints from every nation and from a variety of walks of life – as a form of evangelization in the modern world. His intent was to propose models for contemporary Catholic men and women that they could cherish and, even more important, emulate. Saints are meant primarily to model and to circumscribe the behaviour of the believer, for Catholic teaching holds that all are called to sanctity.

Saint making is therefore an eminently ideological affair, and the trick lies in what sorts of models are being offered up for emulation. An overview of some of the Polish pope's canonizations reveals few surprises: his choices were invariably predictable, offering up models of saintliness that were nothing if not orthodox in both their biographies and their spirituality.

Such models, of course, were exactly what John Paul wanted: they were "safe," in that they embodied the kinds of virtues and values that the church wishes its adherents to follow and to adopt. It was not always like this. Saint making in the early Christian Church was work done by and for the people. Saints were canonized by popular appeal, which did not necessarily guarantee or ensure their respectability. This unpredictability is why the papacy decided that it urgently needed to streamline and control the process. In fact, as more or less practised by the Catholic Church today, formal papal canonization dates only from the early thirteenth century.

In the sociology of sainthood, saints do different things. Apart from the sorts of examples that they suggest and the kinds of behaviours that they are meant to model and therefore to affirm and to control (thereby excluding other less desirable forms of behaviour), they serve as sources of identity. These can be either individual or collective: a personal namesake or a national patron saint. An equally important role has to do – particularly in the Roman Catholic and Orthodox traditions – with the position of the saint as mediator between the earthly and heavenly realms. Saints serve as intercessors. They are the eternal deal makers, hence the historical importance of their relics as tangible evidence of sacred power residing in the here and now.

Young saints, by virtue of their liminal status as children, become particularly "loaded" symbolically. Onto them can be projected any number of adult anxieties, fantasies, and cultural fixations. In their lives, these young saints may have been known for a wide and rather eclectic variety of religious or spiritual disciplines: their humility, their selflessness, their acute sense of mortification, their piety. But what truly set them apart and made them unique – and what really mattered to their sanctity – was ultimately their bodily integrity, their purity. Some maintained it to the end of their young natural lives, whereas others died preserving it. Purity or chastity (also sometimes called virginity, especially in the case of females) became the overarching motif and real raison d'être of youthful sanctity. It was extolled and lauded as a major virtue and a sign of saintly election. One of the more important reasons for this designation was that it marked the young Catholic saint as someone countercultural, someone who "stood squarely against" the prevalent hedonism and impurity of contemporary culture. The chaste teenage saint, of course, was above all exemplary: she or he was meant to inspire Catholic youth to remain on the path of purity. But this chasteness was most definitely gendered: for boys, it meant not indulging in the sin of self-abuse; for girls, it was about maintaining their virginity intact at whatever price. Broader medical and cultural forces were also at work here, especially as regards the understanding of masturbation as both a vice and a disease (Allen 2000, 79-118).

Devotion to these Roman Catholic paragons of chaste youthful sanctity was mediated most effectively through the pedagogical work of a large number of religious teaching orders, both female and male. Through the dedicated care that these nuns, brothers, and priests took in administering and directing the cults of the young saints, a type of sexual pedagogy was created that echoed and strengthened traditional Catholic sexual teaching yet paradoxically also subverted it by proposing alternate models of spiritual and erotic desire (Boisvert 2004). The devotional and pedagogical strategies put in place by the various teaching orders were many and varied. They ran the gamut from school texts, inspirational booklets and leaflets, statues, and holy cards to school plays, clubs, contests, and summer camps. Generally, these can best be classified in terms of a fourfold division: hagiography, iconography, narrative, and pedagogy. Strategies geared to boys were distinct from those geared to girls – strict gender roles remained paramount – but all strategies were embedded in, and thus reflective of, broader concerns with the character and moral or civic development of the young.

In Catholic grammar school, various activities and clubs offered ways for one to build and live a Catholic identity. I remember I had a collection of holy cards of saints, in the same way that other youngsters might collect stamps. These visual tokens of Catholic holy people, many of which had a distinctively tacky religious quality, were meant both to inspire and to reaffirm one's religious belonging. There are even anecdotes of children exchanging them, much as might be done with hockey or baseball cards. I, of course, did not do this; I was more intent on keeping them and on accumulating even more of them when the nuns passed them out for good behaviour. Even then, I knew quite well what a good and proper Catholic boy should be doing with these pious tokens.

Touching Ambivalent and Suffering Bodies
The bodies of young saints are complicated, for sanctity is very much tied up with physicality, as is, of course, sexuality. Anthropological theory reminds us that the human body is a richly charged amalgam of symbols: its disparate parts, including its points of entry and exit, become easily and powerfully loaded with cultural meaning. In Roman Catholicism, particularly at the popular level, the bodies of saints can act as canvases. On them are inscribed – sometimes through strategies of pain and containment, even literally carved – personal and corporate wishes and desires but also orthodox and even less formal forms of belief and devotion. Adolescent saintly bodies remain attractively un- or semi-formed and therefore desiring and erotically emergent bodies – bodies of shame and guilt perhaps but also bodies of wants and needs. In the hagiographic narratives about young saints, there are many subtexts, many complicated levels of interpretation. Their mortal desires, most often transformed into something else, can still be touched beneath the pious words and gestures of the texts

and imagery. When writing about such desires, an exercise of the imagination, a bodily touch across time is called for (Dinshaw 1999).

These young saints were sexually ambiguous icons. The Catholic Church may have tried to put them into neat little boxes labelled "pure and chaste," but like most symbols, particularly human ones, they tended to spill over at the edges. They were multifaceted, erotically charged, and consequently ambiguous. Many came across as rather exotic and attractive androgynous beings. Hagiographic narratives of young holy persons – and the extensive uses to which these were put in the context of Catholic parochial education – often raised troubling sexual questions, many of which, although never fully answered, were strongly hinted at. Language was generally disguised. Sexual desire was part of the stories of these virtuous youngsters but most often in the guise of voyeuristic titillation. Their desires, although couched in the words and imagery of spiritual perfection, were the erotic projections of Catholic adults, whether clerical or lay. It was precisely at this juncture that the chaste teenage saint was manipulated as both impetus and inspiration and that the very real and untamed bodies of flesh and blood Catholic youngsters were transformed into tamed, but no less real or problematic, Catholic bodies. Bodies of pure young saints ultimately held out the promise of Catholic redemption but also of its subversion.

I think of me, the adult scholar of religion and of saints, reaching out across time to try to understand – intellectually touch, as it were – the minds and bodies of these young saints. How can I know what they may have thought, or felt, or even desired? Or should I be concerned with them only as empty cyphers, as virginal templates for the projection of the beliefs and teachings of their clerical guardians? To view them this way would be to undermine their agency, for desire has a marvellous way of seeping through the boundaries that authority likes to draw and fix.

What has happened to me? I have now moved away from my formal Roman Catholic heritage, in large part because of its teachings on a variety of sexual issues, most notably same-sex relations. Yet it was precisely my childhood upbringing in this faith tradition that gave me, I believe, the sensitivity and the ability to accept, to name, and even to celebrate my desires. In this sense, I have subverted the official Catholic narrative. What is truly remarkable is how often I have heard other gay men share a similar story.

There is another type of young saint who, despite not always being viewed at first as a significant model of chasteness or sexual countenance, still raises questions of gender identity in Roman Catholicism. This is the suffering teenage saint, the young holy person who bears physical or mental pain and whose stoicism ultimately is formative of both character and spirituality, which are most often understood as being either feminine or masculine. The sufferings of these holy youth can take several forms: self-imposed mortification or penance; prolonged or life-long illness or other bodily or psychological distress; or acute suffering at the end of life, most often in the case of martyrdom but also due to some type of usually contagious disease. They were expected to die in a particular way and according to a gendered religious script. Although death may have been very far from the minds of most Catholic youth in the first half of the twentieth century, the girls and boys who died in "an aura of sanctity," and who were thus held up as holy models, challenged and inspired these youth to behave like proper Catholic adult men and women.

In my Catholic upbringing, we would occasionally hear of particularly pious youth dying after a long bout of something terrible like tuberculosis. As Sontag (1979) claims in her ground-breaking work on "illness as metaphor," there was a certain romantic quality attached to such ephemeral diseases of the breath. The dying pious youth would be cast in the role of the martyr, and there are stories of some of them having to give up the vocation of a vowed life – especially young boys who wanted to be priests – because they were ill and dying. In these cases, the very act of giving up their dream was seen as contributing to their exceptional sanctity. Such was the story of Gérard Raymond, a Quebec City seminarian who died at the age of nineteen in 1932. In his journal, he wrote of his fervent desire to die as a martyred missionary priest. French Canadian mothers would often cite his pious and ascetic life as an inspiration for their wayward sons.

In the pantheon of Roman Catholic holy youth, St. Maria Goretti (1890-1902) and St. Dominic Savio (1842-57) represent ideal types. At the time of their canonizations, each was hailed by the Vatican as a particularly apt and inspiring model for Catholic youth to follow. Each also emerges as a rather complex and charged symbol, far more multilayered than might be assumed or expected. In the case of Goretti, much has been written about how her attempted rape and subsequent murder (she was canonized not as a martyr for the faith but as a martyr for purity, the first such case) became a powerful and ultimately problematic and damaging source of sexual identity and anxiety for Catholic girls. As for Savio, he was a student of one of the largest and most influential Catholic male teaching orders, the Salesians, and his cult, still in effect today, has taken a variety of disparate and interesting directions that reflect changes in the church's approach to, and understanding of, adolescent psychology. These young Italian saints became, in the first half of the twentieth century, two of the most influential pedagogical models of bodily integrity and moral uprightness for Roman Catholic youth, and their life stories served as clarion calls for a distinctively countercultural Catholic sexual morality.

In my youth – for I too attended a Salesian school – I had a particular fascination with, and a devotion to, Dominic Savio. In one text, I even call him "my boyfriend." The priests and brothers may have wanted to put him forth as a model of perfect purity and obedience, but I responded much more subversively to him as a source of emerging same-sex desire. Savio became for me, as it were, the means through which I was able to hold in some delicate balance two identities: a religious one, particularly my early sense of a calling to the priesthood, and a nascent sexual one. In this way, he became an "instrument of formation" but certainly not in the ways that the Salesians, in their inspired naïveté, were intending or even imagining.

The "Maria Goretti" Paradigm

Maria Goretti was a twelve-year-old Italian peasant girl who died in 1902 after being stabbed repeatedly for refusing to submit to the sexual advances of a nineteen-year-old farmhand, whom she forgave on her deathbed. She was canonized by Pius XII in 1950, at a time when a more permissive secular youth culture was coming into its own in the West. Maria Goretti became the ideal Catholic saint for young girls, who were strongly encouraged to be like her, even to the point of death, in defending their bodily integrity. As mentioned previously, she was the first female martyr to be canonized not because she had died for the faith, as was the case with saints of the early church, but because she had fought for her virginity and saved it – a clear indication of the worth of chastity and purity as desirable and legitimate Catholic values, especially during that supposedly dangerous period of life known as adolescence. In the modern era, Maria Goretti stands as the paradigmatic young, female Catholic saint, and her short life and macabre death provide the script for other holy tales of young(ish) and equally heroic virgins. In fact, the Catholic Church turned her into an intensely "sexualized" saint.

In the 1950s and 1960s, Maria Goretti became a bit of a Catholic cottage industry. Her story attracted sensationalistic, heroic, misogynistic, and sexually repressive readings. In North America she became somewhat of a middle-class saint, embodying middle-class sexual norms and expectations for young girls (Norris 1996). Her image was omnipresent in Catholic girls' schools, and her life was often used by nuns as a type of sexual pedagogy for their young charges. Maria has been interpreted, in turn, as a model of penitence and obedience, of a properly devoted family life, of bourgeois respectability, of the romance and spiritual innocence of peasant society, of the Catholic response to attempted rape, of Christian forgiveness, and of female naïveté. She has also been a source of bawdy religious and ethnic humour. One could say that this is a great deal of responsibility to put on the shoulders of a twelve-year-old girl, as saintly as she may have been. What is the meaning of each of these spins on Maria Goretti's story, and why was there a need to do any "spinning" in the first place? What does it mean that a young and devout Italian peasant girl from the nineteenth century should be used to instruct a North American Catholic girl of the mid-twentieth on how to respect her body? How does this adolescent girl "read" the life, but most especially the violent death, of Maria Goretti: with reverence or with a good dose of youthful impudence? And how does the scholar, in turn, "read" the adolescent "reading" the saint? Her holy tale – part fact, part fiction – has been used and reused in the service of a multiplicity of agendas, including, quite naturally, those of the Catholic Church itself.

In fact, much of the hagiographic material about Maria Goretti, including that written by clergy, is marked by a strong sense of voyeuristic titillation. This is not unusual in writings devoted to the stories of young female saints. These stories are meant to be moral tales, and they are designed to serve cautionary ends. Part of their discursive strategy involves the hinting at – and sometimes the outright displaying of – lurid erotic details, making them more akin to soft porn than to traditional devotional literature. These stories are purposely meant to enflame the male gaze, the better ultimately to demonize it. In these tales, it is most often the young saint herself who stands in as the source of temptation: her virginity and purity are sources of erotic attraction for the bestial male, who somehow cannot help giving himself over to his baser passions. The saint occupies a strategically liminal, mixed state: she is an object both of attraction and repulsion. It is her shaming that ultimately resolves the erotic tension, a tension that is really and ultimately male-centred.

Norris (1996, 223), in her insightful essay on Maria Goretti, asks whether she was "cipher or saint." The answer, we know, is tied up with the male gaze. It is men who so often do the looking, in every sense of the word. It is they who, by virtue of privilege and authority, get to circumscribe the discourse, and it is they who get to dissect and label the saintly female body in its component parts. It is men, after all, who canonize, who ultimately get to sanction orthodoxy. The female saint is reduced to the female body, a fact that only plays further into patriarchal discourse. In many ways, this is exactly what happened to Maria Goretti. She *did* become a cipher: an "empty" person defined by nothing more than her intact virginity, a template by and through which were read and defined – indeed, controlled – the virginal bodies of other Catholic girls. The overriding, violent, sadistic message was always and everywhere one and the same: better death than sin, better savage violence than loss of purity, better sanctity than defilement. For the Catholic Church, this was the stark choice that every young girl might be called upon to make.

At the heart of every female virgin saint's story – that of St. Maria Goretti or any of the countless others – stands one incontrovertible fact, one dynamic: that of power. It comes in different guises, and it can be spoken by different players in the drama. It can most certainly be the voice of masculine authority asserting patriarchal power over chaste or unmarried female flesh, very often to the point of attempted rape or physical violence. It can equally be the cold, confident gaze of the saint herself speaking "no" to this power, thereby claiming authority and integrity for herself, choosing being over nonbeing. It can be the official power of a churchly male voice raising certain models of submissive femaleness to the glories of the altar. Or it can be these models redefined and reappropriated in all their hidden power: women of character and fortitude who have gone where no man has gone before. The saintly female body can become a model for other, more "ordinary" female bodies. Norris (1996, 192) observes,

> For Maria Goretti, the issue was not a roll in the hay. The loss of her virginity in a rigidly patriarchal peasant culture could have had economic and social consequences so dire that it might well have seemed a choice between being and non-being. And is it foolish for a girl to have such a strong sense of her self that she resists its violation, resists being asked to do, in the private spaces of her body, what she does not want to do?

Norris's question effectively turns the traditional Maria Goretti melodrama on its head, although it does not really do away with the thread of clerical misogyny that has sustained this melodrama.

As late as the 1980s, the Catholic Church was still proposing the Maria Goretti saintly ideal of purity as appropriate for Catholic women. In October 1987 Pope John Paul II beatified another slightly older Italian "martyr for purity," Blessed Pierina Morosini, who died while defending her virginity against a twenty-year-old attacker. She had picked up a stone to protect herself, but the man used it to strike her on the head, and she died from the wounds. Morosini had attended the beatification of Maria Goretti as a pilgrim in Rome in 1947, where she was reputed to have said that she wanted to die like the new martyr. Maria Goretti provided a model of holy femaleness for Morosini to emulate and was most certainly a saintly guide and protector to her, someone who helped Morosini to make sense of the final, most traumatic act of her life. Through the heroics of the story, however, the interests of the male church are once again upheld; it is the virginal female body, not the sexually knowledgeable one, that receives the exaltation and glory of sainthood. In fact, one of the recurring criticisms of female canonizations under John Paul II was that he repeated and reinforced this traditional equation of virginity with sanctity and did not propose models with which modern married women could identify.

Maintaining the Maria Goretti paradigm of female sanctity effectively allows the Roman Catholic Church to keep "problematic" female flesh at bay by idealizing, sanctifying, and glorifying it – and thereby erasing it. This is perhaps the most insidious part of all, for at the centre of these hagiographic stories of attempted rape of Maria and so many other young female saints – even into the contemporary era – lies one hard, cold, and unmistakable message: better to be a "whole" woman, even dead, than a partially defiled one because therein lies the path to sanctity. Flesh and blood female lives do not truly count in this equation. The saint herself is here understood as serving a larger, more altruistic purpose. Her death becomes the means by which others are saved, often the men who did them violence. The young virginal saint then truly becomes a cipher, and her martyrdom, with its attendant violence, becomes a path of redemption for someone else. The existence of the saint, her body, her suffering, her innocence, her future – all are "relativized" in the service of some higher, more noble goal. The saint essentially becomes expendable, most often in the interests of the male's hegemony and, ultimately, his redemption. It could be argued that the younger the saint, the more she is seen as being superfluous to the moral of the story. There is something slightly pornographic in this: the man's satisfaction is what ultimately counts.

It is the theological and hagiographic "covering and uncovering" of these saintly female bodies that causes a problem. Their virginity, although hidden, is continuously being shown in public, and it is invariably displayed through the normative prism of male desire. These young virginal women, as saintly as they may be, become the "other" in that they are covered and uncovered simultaneously – exotic yet familiar, secret yet exposed, erotic yet sacred, pure yet potentially tainted. The question can be asked: purity for the sake of what, and of whom? Here, the answer cuts one way, no doubt, for the prurient theological and educational interests of a celibate male church but also – and perhaps primarily – another way for the young holy women themselves and others like them.

As problematic and devastating as saintly models may be in controlling and channelling the behaviour, needs, and aspirations of the Catholic faithful, saints can also serve as empowering models subversive of orthodoxy. Saints don't always do what the church tells them to do. They are often deliberately and creatively used by their devotees to serve subversive stratagems. St. Maria Goretti and her heavenly companions may well seek to limit and control a young girl's sexual options, but they also give her power: the power of refusal, the power of being. These saintly virgins make possible a sacred space and time to speak a definitive "no" to male sexual hegemony and power. But as Norris (1996, 192) suggests, this speaking happens only in "the private spaces of her body," not because the church may have said the young woman has no other choice and certainly not because, from the perspective of the institutional church, death is superior to the loss of bodily integrity. Saying "no" does not, need not, and should not imply death. The church may have imprinted Maria Goretti's "no" on the malleable young bodies of countless generations of older Catholic women – and they may have resented its imposition – but this "no," in fact, may have kept them whole. The bodies of Catholic children, it was thought – especially those of Catholic girls – needed to be policed and disciplined. The times have not really changed all that much. The Catholic Church is still rallying pure heavenly bodies in its ongoing battle against human bodily desire. Catholic discourses of youthful female sexuality in the mid- and late twentieth century bear a saintly imprimatur. Such an imprimatur certainly regulates, prohibits, manipulates, and denies, yet can it also liberate, subvert, affirm, and elevate?

The "Dominic Savio" Ideal

Dominic Savio was born in the Piedmont region of northern Italy on 2 April 1842, the son of a blacksmith and the second child of a family of ten. From the beginning, his health was frail, yet he harboured a persistent desire to become a priest. The home environment was a religious one, and Dominic is reputed to have been particularly pious from an early age. He received his first communion when he was only seven years old, a highly unusual practice for the time. Among the resolutions he took on this day, "Death, but not sin" remains, by far, the most significant in terms of his subsequent spiritual development. In his life of Savio, St. John Bosco relates an incident at the age of ten when companions of the young boy pleaded with him to go bathing with them at a swimming hole in the heat of summer, presumably naked. Dominic, as might be expected, steadfastly refused, claiming that it constituted an occasion of sin. Bosco's (1996, 38) commentary on the event is especially telling: "How many youngsters mourn the loss of their innocence and attribute the reason to having gone bathing with such lads in those unfortunate places?" One is not sure exactly what might have happened, but the tale fixes the virtue of purity at the very centre of the young boy's personality and future sanctity. At the age of twelve, Dominic entered the Oratory of St. Francis de Sales in Turin, thereby coming under the direct tutelage of Bosco himself, who had founded the school and its religious order, the Salesians, some eight years earlier. It was in large part based on his three short years at the oratory that the young Dominic's reputation for sanctity was established.

Dominic's life at the oratory was that of an ordinary student, although it was marked by an acute sense of piety, obedience, and devotion to the rules and by a confident zeal in caring for the religious welfare of his schoolmates. The young boy was also keen on engaging in extreme forms of bodily mortification, but Bosco forbade it on the grounds of his age and poor health. Among the mundane incidents that later became the stuff of hagiographic legend, one particularly famous story revolves around a violent stone fight that Dominic interrupted by placing himself between the two protagonists, raised crucifix in hand, and asking them to kill him instead of each other. Other stories tell of the young saint being found in a state of ecstasy in the chapel; of his angrily tearing up a dirty magazine that his companions were laughing at; of prophecies and dreams concerning the state of the Catholic Church in England and the future of the Salesian order; and even of a vision about curing his own sick mother. In February 1857, due to deteriorating health and an inflammation of the lungs (tuberculosis), he was sent home. Bled to excess, he died, apparently in rapture, on 9 March, a few weeks short of his fifteenth birthday. Dominic Savio was canonized in 1954.

John Bosco's philosophy of education was progressive for the time. At the height of the Industrial Revolution in northern Italy, he had noticed that young boys, most often from the countryside, found themselves homeless and adrift in the urban squalor of Turin. He decided to devote himself to their welfare, believing that, by recreating as normal a home life as possible at the oratory, he could save them from the worst spiritual and material ravages of their precarious existence. Education was then considered a bourgeois privilege, certainly not something for the poor or the working classes. He also espoused the teaching of trades to equip the youth with employable skills.

At the oratory, Bosco emphasized a number of principles in the education of the boys: cheerfulness, leadership, piety (but not to excess), and most important, the control over the senses that was needed to avoid occasions of sin. The latter was often understood to refer to the ideal of bodily purity. When he wrote the life of Dominic Savio some years later, these were the same virtues and qualities that he portrayed the young saint as possessing to an extraordinary degree. Savio thus became the ideal Salesian boy, the very model that *all* boys in *all* Salesian schools should emulate and to which they could turn for strength in fighting their own all-too-human battles for spiritual perfection. Ultimately, the virtues that St. Dominic Savio had lived by, especially that of chastity, were those that *all* Catholic boys should copy.

Nonetheless, much ambivalence surrounds the virtuous Dominic Savio. As one reads Bosco's life of the youth, one is struck by the fact that Savio is so often portrayed as an angelic youth – as rather prissy, in fact – although Bosco goes to great lengths to assure his readers that the emerging saint was very much a boy like all the others, if perhaps less rowdy. There are even hints of some "special friendships" between Dominic and two other schoolmates with whom he was especially close. Although nothing sexual is implied, the tone of the text, when read for its ambiguities, does leave certain possibilities open. In the iconography of the young saint (statues, holy cards, and so forth), his most striking feature is his androgynous look. This is not unrelated to the fact that the Salesians themselves chose to portray Savio, both visually and pedagogically, as a somewhat effeminate, virginal child. Dominic Savio's ambivalence as the perfect and chaste youth – yet suspect because of his androgyny – makes him susceptible to certain forms of projection. Consider how a sexually confused, young gay boy might respond to Dominic Savio, quite apart from the obviously religious aspects of the devotion to him as a saint. Desire is not foreign to sanctity; it may, in fact, be one of sanctity's most attractive qualities.

Salesian discourse about Dominic Savio was clearly consistent with what the order understood to be its primary educational mission in the church: the formation of virtuous young men. "Virtuous" could mean many things – obedient, generous, pious, even cheerful of heart – but it implied being pure above all. And for young adolescents, this implication was clear: be chaste in mind *and* body; above all, be wary of that most serious and destructive of all sins, the solitary one. Enter St. Dominic Savio, the chaste and innocent one, the perfect boy. At Salesian schools, orphanages, summer camps, and other such educational institutions the world over, his angelic face and heroic virtue were supposed to keep Salesian boys under control, metaphorically and literally. Savio clubs, whose primary purpose was to encourage imitation of the young saint in all things, sprang up. His feast day on 9 March was an occasion for public ceremonials and contests of all sorts. His statue and image looked down serenely from Salesian walls, overseeing the preservation of manly Salesian virtues, especially that of youthful purity. This purity was his prized treasure, his true mark of greatness, his lasting legacy.

When I was a youngster, I read a lot of stories about saints' lives. Some of these accounts could be quite lurid, like the text of Maria Goretti's life, which was more a turn-on because of the depiction of the swarthy farmhand than an incitement to pious emulation. Others, like Dominic Savio's story, carried me away in an exalted mood of adventure and romance. I too wanted to be a saint like these young heroes, even if this was ultimately an unpopular career choice. I was also a young boy struggling with an emerging sense of sexual difference. Saints' stories normalized this difference. Their queer, non-normative lives mirrored and revalued my own.

Some Points of Convergence

I offer three points of convergence – three open questions – that may help to situate this discussion of young Roman Catholic saints within the broader focus of how sexuality and gender can become significant "flash points" for religious institutions. First, it must be noted that the topic of youth and sexuality, particularly in religious institutions but also in culture more generally, has always been a deeply contested site of interpretation and conflict, even more so in our present day (see Shipley, Chapter 4, this volume). So the question is: do stories of pure young saints ultimately offer a safer and more hidden – because ultimately more theologically orthodox – means of dealing with this sensitive issue? Or do they instead further expose and dilute it? Second, given the crisis of abuse now confronting the Roman Catholic Church, the question can legitimately be asked: how might notions and images of glorified young holy bodies have played into the sorts of behaviours that were seen as being legitimized and encouraged? In other words, did these young saints and their pure lives contribute to an overall understanding of "holy" young bodies as being sexually and morally available to "consecrated" older bodies? Third, it is obvious that a Catholic sexual pedagogy was created through the stories and images of these young saints – one that has had a determining influence on generations of practising Catholics, many of whom have responded by leaving the church. So the question is: did this Catholic sexual pedagogy ultimately carry the seeds of its own institutional diminishment and disaffiliation? In a world where religion has become ever more urgently the focus of tension and cultural anxiety, these questions warrant serious engagement. They compel and summon us to a place of renewed reflection.

Note
Research for this chapter was supported by a grant from the Social Sciences and Humanities Research Council of Canada.

References
Allen, P.L. 2000. *The Wages of Sin: Sex and Disease, Past and Present*. Chicago: University of Chicago Press.
Boisvert, D.L. 2004. *Sanctity and Male Desire: A Gay Reading of Saints*. Cleveland: Pilgrim.
Bosco, J. 1996. *The Life of Saint Dominic Savio*. New Rochelle, NY: Salesiana.
Castelli, E.A. 2004. *Martyrdom and Memory: Early Christian Culture Making*. New York: Columbia University Press.
Dinshaw, C. 1999. *Getting Medieval: Sexualities and Communities, Pre- and Postmodern*. Durham, NC: Duke University Press.
Norris, K. 1996. *The Cloister Walk*. New York: Riverhead Books.
Orsi, R.A. 2005. *Between Heaven and Earth: The Religious Worlds People Make and the Scholars Who Study Them*. Princeton, NJ: Princeton University Press.
Sontag, S. 1979. *Illness as Metaphor*. New York: Vintage.

8

Corporeal Diversity in the Religion of Sport
THE DEBATE OVER ENHANCED BODIES

Tracy J. Trothen

South African runner Oscar Pistorius adorned posters and other advertisements for the London 2012 Olympic Games. He was born without fibulae, and both legs were amputated below the knee when he was eleven months old. Prostheses have since allowed him to walk and run. Controversy regarding Pistorius's "Cheetah legs" did not begin until he applied to compete in the Olympics. The runner's prostheses are high-tech, carbon-fibre prosthetics that, according to some experts, unfairly advantage Pistorius over able-bodied athletes (Burkett, McNamee and Potthast 2011; Sutcliffe 2008). These studies contributed to the January 2008 decision of the International Association of Athletics Federation (IAAF) to ban Pistorius from its competitions, including the Olympics. Later in 2008 the Court of Arbitration for Sport overturned this decision and approved Pistorius for Olympic competition, concluding that his prostheses did not give him an overall advantage (Burkett, McNamee, and Potthast 2011). Although he did not qualify for the 2008 Games, on 23 March 2011 Pistorius made the qualifying time for the 400-metre race and the 400-metre relay, leaving it up to the South African Olympic Association to decide whether he would compete in the 2012 Games (Davies 2011). Pistorius competed in the 2012 London Summer Olympics but did not medal. Technological innovation had made it possible for Pistorius to run and successfully compete in the Paralympics. His Cheetah legs, his drive to compete, and a systemic valuing of the "normal" Olympics (Swartz and Watermeyer 2008) subsequently led to Pistorius's application to IAAF competitions, including the Olympics. Pistorius's visible differentness has generated controversy, confusion, and intrigue.

Many recognized religions, as is evidenced throughout this volume, avoid, deny, or otherwise negate human embodiment. This failure of religion, particularly much of Euro-American Christianity, to engage sufficiently with embodiment has left unchallenged normative values that exclude and often penalize those who do not visibly fit within sexual norms. These values privilege those who appear to fit as clearly male or female (in spite of the scientific knowledge that there are multiple sex categories), and entwined with these two sex categories are expectations regarding acceptable sexual desire (e.g., heterosexual) and practice.

Embodiment necessarily includes sexuality. And sexuality includes but is more than genital sex. As contemporary researchers have noted,[1]

> The literature of sexual theology or embodiment theology ... has suggested that sexuality is much more of an integral and holistic part of the human experience than the activity of genital sex. It is the source of our capacity for relationship, for emotional and erotic connection, for intimacy, for passion and for transcendence. It is a holistic expression of our human experience as *body-selves*.[2] (Horn et al. 2005, 81-82, emphasis in original)

This chapter builds on the body of scholarship linking identity categories related to embodiment – including sex, gender, race, and ability or disability – with sexual practice and desire (e.g., Foucault 1979; Butler 1990; Shogan 1999; Isherwood 2000; Stuart 2000).

In the 1970s and 1980s, North American feminism drew a distinction between sex and gender as a way to underscore the relevance of social construction and to challenge essentialist understandings of gender. Since then, it has become increasingly clear that not only are notions of gender at least in part socially constructed and unstable, but so too are notions of sex.[3] According to medical science, many people do not fit into the sex categories of male or female. Further, characteristics deemed masculine (e.g., muscular limbs or facial hair) or feminine (e.g., slim upper body or wide hips) can appear on any body. Despite this diversity, and in some sense because of it, the assumption that sex, gender, sexual desire, and practice are tied together in predictable ways persists: men are masculine, sexually desire women, and have sexual intercourse with women (Shogan 1999, 56-63). Similarly, women are feminine, sexually desire men, and have sexual intercourse with men. It is often presumed that the meanings of femininity and masculinity are directly connected to how one practices sex; women are passive and penetrable, whereas men are aggressive and penetrating.

Elite sport has long been a cultural area dominated by the masculine and heterosexual norm (e.g., Shogan 1999, 61; Stebner and Trothen 2002). Women and stereotypically gay men visibly disrupt this norm. This disruption is intensified, for example, by female athletes who appear even more muscular than the average or by male distance runners who appear even slimmer and less muscular in their upper bodies than what is assumed to be average. The study of embodiment in elite sport implicitly addresses these associations and norms regarding sexuality. Sport is an important socio-cultural location for embodiment, including sexuality, as sport paradoxically is built around maintaining embodiment norms and transcending embodiment limitations. For those whose embodied identities do not "fit," sport is a venue where they have variously found a home or experienced further pressure to conform (Bridel and Rail 2007; Ravel and Rail 2008; Shogan 1999).

Not only is sport both a locus for exceptional embodiment and a social force in the propagation of values regarding embodiment diversity, but increasingly scholars are also establishing a link between sport and religion, arguing variably that sport is a type of religion, is similar to religion, or is associated with religion. As a secular religion, sport is centred on the body as a source of wonder and possible transcendence. Through the lens of the enhancement debate that has dominated elite sport, this chapter examines the treatment and transformative potential of embodiment diversity within the secular religion of sport.

Elite athletics represents a secular religion that is global and mainstream. This secular religion showcases a range of fit bodies, establishing rules for acceptable embodiment diversity. Science is challenging these rules with the creation of technologies that are changing and revealing bodies. This interfacing of elite sport with techno-science brings into focus what are considered acceptable, desirable, and ideal bodies. The exploration of four main approaches to the enhancement debate provides a window into how embodiment diversity is regarded in elite sport. This exploration illumines the moral relevance of socially normative values to elite sport's approach to embodiment diversity. The focus within the enhancement debate on acceptability has led away from intentional critiques of these normative values and epistemologies. Not only has this focus been unsuccessful in terms of constructing clear criteria for the assessment of advantages, but it has also camouflaged larger underlying issues, including what is valuable about corporeal personhood and sport.

I approach this topic as a social ethicist drawing on postmodernism. Accordingly, I am interested in exposing causal dynamics, particularly operative values. Often we assume that an issue can be seen in only one or a limited number of ways. This is largely due to a failure to see that existing approaches assume particular values and ways of viewing the world. As Kahane (2011, 355) observes, "recent philosophy has neglected important questions about value – questions that are not about well-being, autonomy or justice but about what attitude we should have to the world and our place in it." When questions are asked about the values that are attached to ways of seeing the enhancement issue, it becomes clear that the debate would be shaped differently if alternative, more marginalized values informed the approaches taken.

Several European philosophers have argued that technology is not value-neutral but inculcates values of efficiency and utility (Marcuse 1964; Habermas 1968; Foucault 1988). Neither is elite sport value-neutral; winning and the economic and political fruits that follow drive a significant part of elite sport (e.g., Simon 2004; van Hilvoorde, Vos, and de Wert 2007). The uncritical absorption of the technological values of efficiency and utility may have a doubling effect on the reduction of elite sport to winning. However, as recreational sport suggests, it is possible to cultivate other, more marginalized values such as diversity and the pleasure of playing the game, or competing intensely, regardless of outcome. These values do exist in elite sport, but they are not normative. In using a social ethics approach to analyze the controversy over the use of enhancement techno-science in sport, I ask what assumptions and values have shaped this ethical debate (Legge 2006).

Insights from postmodernism about the dangers of epistemological assumptions and generalizations are very useful to this chapter. As theological ethicist Ivone Gebara (2002, 73) notes, all "epistemology can be seen as ethics, and all ethics is epistemology." This perspective emphasizes the centrality of how we know to the discipline of ethics. Questions such as whose interests are served by the ways that knowledge is constructed reveal values that inform how we think about the world.

Assumptions and values shape epistemological categories of embodiment. These categories are often binary and include male and female, abled and disabled, and homosexual and heterosexual. Fault lines are exposed when people do not "fit" these categories. The sport enhancement debate is making more visible the fault lines in normative constructions of embodiment (Davey 2002; Jönsson 2007). For example, media coverage of an extremely physically fit and often sweat-covered Pistorius imparts very sexualized images that disrupt the expectation that people who are defined as physically disabled are asexual (Stuart 2000). People rarely fit static or essentialist categories; rather, identities are delightfully fluid and unstable (King 2008). However, as will become evident, in elite sport the points of disjuncture with commonly accepted epistemological categories tend to be glossed over (thus preserving the normative order) unless these differences are too visible.

The exposure of the fault lines in normative ways of knowing can be dramatic when the person is a high-profile athlete. As far as sporting events go, the Olympics are the clearest example of a global event that attracts huge corporate and political interest groups. When an Olympic athlete such as "Blade Runner" Oscar Pistorius disrupts normative categories, much attention is generated. As will become clear, when this disruption concerns embodiment norms and, with those norms, expectations regarding gender and sexuality, the level of attention and controversy is magnified. How this embodiment diversity is regarded in the secular religion of elite sport is the subject of this chapter. My intent is to generate more questions through reflection on the ethical complexity of the intersection of enhancement options, embodiment diversity, religion, and sport.

Similar to the methodologies used by other authors in this volume, including Catherine Holtmann, Nancy Nason-Clark, and Andrew Kam-Tuk Yip, I introduce partial narratives of particular elite athletes throughout the chapter to illustrate the relevance of the sport enhancement debate to religious and embodiment diversity.

Religion and Sport

Some organized religions, particularly in North America, are seeing their followings decrease as people find alternate ways and places in which to express their spiritualities.[4] Sport is a significant example of such an alternate space.

Sport, it has been claimed, is a religion (Prebish 1993), a civil religion (Bellah 1967), a popular religion (Price 2001), a folk religion (Mathisen 2001), a natural religion (Novak 1993), a cultural religion (Albanese 1982), a form of lived religion (Sanford 2007, 888), a way of being religious (Sinclair-Faulkner 1977), sometimes a spiritual discipline (Trothen 2006; Austin 2010), or a type of evangelism in the case of modern "muscular Christianity" (Ladd and Mathisen 1999). The questions of whether sport is a religion and, if so, what type of religion are debated. However, most agree that many features of sport have religious-like overtones, such as pregame processionals, the similarity between star players and gods or goddesses, the parallels between commentators and scribes, the resemblance between trophies and icons (Price 2001), and the sense of transcendence or flow reported by participants and followers (Jackson and Csikszentmihalyi 1999; Kelly 2011; Martinkova and Parry 2011).

As religious studies scholar A. Whitney Sanford (2007, 888) observes, although debates continue about whether or how the sacred is "truly" experienced in sport, "many [sports] participants ... understand their experience as sacred, spiritual, or religious, and broadening our definitions of religion to recognize these experiences as religious is a step toward recognizing the self-declared religious practices of many North Americans." Similarly, drawing on his field research on college football in the southern United States, Eric Bain-Selbo (2009) concludes that college football functions religiously for many fans and players. Self-described religious-like or spiritual experiences in sport are important to recognize. It is also important to realize that sport does not have an exclusive claim on such bodily spiritual experiences. Others have similarly understood dance, music, or art (e.g., Callaway 2013). A notable feature of sport is the vast numbers of followers/viewers, particularly for elite levels. In North America one thinks of the Olympics, Super Bowl Sunday, and particularly for Canadians, the Stanley Cup Finals.

One aspect of this secular religion is what athletes often refer to as a sense of transcendence or flow (Jackson and Csikszentmihalyi 1999; Kelly 2011; Martinkova and Parry 2011). This experience in sport usually occurs in the midst of intense absorption, embodiment, and exertion, when everything else is cleared away and a deep sense of connectedness and effortlessness emerges (Sanford 2007). As a distance runner in a study by Susan Jackson and Mihalyi Csikszentmihalyi (1999, 75) describes it, "You are going faster, and yet it seems easier ... It is hard to describe in words unless you experience it ... You're going as fast as you can go, and yet you're doing it quite easily." Using theological terms, religious studies scholar Lawrence W. Fagg (2003, 560) calls this the "seamless continuum" between experiences of transcendence and immanence (see also Moltmann 1985, 15; and Moltmann 1992). These moments of transcendence through immanence defy a separation between the sacred and the profane.

By locating the sacred in the physical, one queers or makes strange (King 2008) the normative Western Christian assumption that the sacred is restricted to the spirit and thus excludes the material or physical. Sport as a secular religion denies not only the sacred-profane bifurcation (Moltmann 1992; Dickey Young 2002; Lynch 2007; Sanford 2007; for a more in-depth deconstruction of this bifurcation, see also Holtmann, Chapter 6, this volume) but also the related immanent-transcendent binary (Trothen 2012). In other words, the sacred is often experienced as something profoundly holy and more than humans can know (transcendent), yet this knowledge is almost paradoxically generated through embodiment (immanent); sport shows that the transcendent can be experienced through the immanent and that the sacred can be touched through the profane.

Sport's focus on embodiment makes its way of experiencing the sacred very different from that of more normative Western religious traditions. This is not to say that there are not other ways of experiencing the sacred that focus on embodiment but only that sport is one such way. Finally, by locating the sacred within embodiment, sport disrupts epistemological presumptions, categories, and normative values. In particular, embodiment is not experienced as separate from the sacred but is instead the vehicle for touching the sacred. The religion of sport celebrates embodiment.

However, questions remain about the acceptable range of this embodiment. This concern with limits has been the focus of the enhancement debate.

Sport and Enhancement Techno-Science

The sport enhancement debate, I contend, is more appropriately understood as an embodiment diversity debate that includes added so-called enhancements. When the debate is limited to one of "enhancement," it is framed by the assumption that this issue concerns only added enhancing interventions. The issue is more comprehensive. Science is showing us that many factors influence and change bodies. Some elite athletes such as cyclist Lance Armstrong have been caught cheating by using prohibited "doping" substances such as anabolic steroids and exogenous erythropoietin (EPO). As the enhancement options increase through innovations in technology, the cognitive sciences, robotics, genetic modification technologies, cybernetics, and other fields, it is important to ask why some advantages are deemed fair and others not. Embodiment advantages include motivational music, sports psychology techniques, meditation and prayer ("emotional doping"), prosthetic devices ("technological doping"), polyurethane swimsuits ("doping-on-a-hanger"), genetic modification technologies ("gene doping"), vitamins, and hypobaric chambers, in addition to just plain doping (e.g., anabolic steroids and blood doping). Advantages deemed unacceptable are often referred to pejoratively as "doping." This labelling limits constructive debate by asserting that these advantages are morally bad.

Genetic modification technologies pose particularly important questions. For example, what will happen in the future when an athlete is born with genetic advantages as a result of a parent or grandparent making a decision to use germ-line genetic modification technologies (Miah 2004; Trothen 2009)? Will this person be considered to have an unacceptable or a natural advantage? Is it not ethically problematic to make a choice that will affect future generations without their consent? An infamous example of an emergent genetic modification technology of interest in elite sport is Repoxygen. This gene therapy increases EPO, causing an increase in red blood cells and thus oxygen capacity, which enhances endurance. Such technology would be of interest to endurance sports such as long-distance running, skiing, and cycling. In 2006 Thomas Springstein, a German track coach was found guilty of trying to procure Repoxygen for his athletes (Aschwanden 2012). Although athletes who are born with impressive aerobic capacities are perceived to be lucky, the use of genetic modification technologies continues to be unacceptable. The question at the core of the enhancement debate has been which advantages are acceptable. This question, I will show, is not only problematic but also inadequate, for it fails to address underlying questions about values and meaning.

While additional enhancing options are becoming available, science is also revealing the vast diversity among existing human embodiment through such techniques as magnetic resonance imaging, genetic analysis and profiling, medical lab tests, and interdisciplinary "gender testing." Through these means, many hitherto unproven and, sometimes, unsuspected advantages are made visible. South African runner Caster Semenya garnered unwanted attention by winning the women's 800-metre race at the 2009 IAAF World Championships in Athletics. The problem was that she won it by a pronounced margin of 2.45 seconds. Because the margin was so wide and because many thought she had "masculine" features, it was speculated that Semenya was a man.[5] Semenya was subjected to gender testing and rumoured to have "failed" these tests. After an eleven-month suspension, it was announced that she could return to competition (Vannini and Fornssler 2010). Due to confidentiality, the results of the test remain unknown; it is possible that she was required to undergo hormone therapy. The use of science to determine whether Semenya qualified for the category of woman raises a number of important questions about embodiment diversity and normative values. For example, females are expected to be pretty, whereas males are to be muscular (Ratele 2011). When people do not fit well into these values and categories, especially if such people are in the media spotlight, controversy follows. In the case of elite sport, the critique is usually framed in terms of unfair advantage.

Science is showing that there is more embodiment diversity than has been presumed. Not only are variations in narrowly construed gender and sex constructions (Shogan 1999, 60) becoming more known (as are the implications of this diversity for athletic competition), but science is also making visible the physiological advantages created through the use of media such as music, meditation, and prayer. In 2007 the *New York Times* reported that USA Track and Field, the body that governs running in the United States, had "banned the use of headphones and portable audio players like iPods at its official races ... to ensure safety and to prevent runners from having a competitive edge" (Macur 2007; see also Nowotny and Testa 2010). Although this ruling proved impractical to enforce, the suggestion that iPods are a form of emotional doping is yet another example of how science and technology are not only improving sporting enhancements but also making visible the array of competitive edges.

Other such advantages that science is making increasingly difficult to ignore are those from the genetic lottery. More of these by-chance enhancements are becoming easily detectable. For example, aerobic capacity can be determined, as can one's genetic ability to improve this capacity with training (Bouchard 2012). The anticipated science of genetic "signatures" (i.e., the nucleotide sequences that are specific to an individual) will reveal more such advantages, or so-called "anomalies" (Friedmann 2012). This science will also provide a means of detecting "gene doping," which is the use of genetic modification technologies to enhance athletic performance. Currently, the use of genetic modification technologies is undetectable except through invasive muscle biopsies (McCrory 2003). Genetic signatures will also make existing embodiment diversity more visible by showing what advantages individual athletes might possess in their genes.

Adequate approaches to the sport enhancement debate must take into account this array of advantages: the visible, invisible, added, and by-chance.

Approaches to the Sport Enhancement Debate

There have been four main approaches to the sport enhancement debate; all are concerned primarily with establishing criteria for assessing which enhancements are acceptable. Such approaches miss the relevance of techno-science that makes existing advantages visible. These approaches also tend to be uncritical of elite sport's normative values, including the emphasis on winning, efficiency, status, and money, and tend to accept its corresponding neglect of beauty, wonder, diversity, and the playing of the game. This does not mean that these latter values are not important to some athletes and others in elite sport or that winning and these latter values are mutually exclusive.

The four main approaches to the sport enhancement debate rely on the following, not undisputed, criteria for assessing the acceptability of an enhancement: (1) whether it is judged natural (good) or artificial (bad), (2) whether it is the individual athlete's choice (assuming that it has not been judged to pose health risks); (3) whether it is judged to be fair in competition; and (4) whether it unduly compromises the internal goods of (the) sport. Most approaches emphasize one of these but may additionally employ the other criteria. Each approach is explored below in terms of its relevance to embodiment diversity.

Enhancements as Natural (Good) or Artificial (Bad)

Distinguishing between natural and artificial is problematic. These concepts are unstable, and the divide between them rests on the constructed concept of "normal." Further complicating this approach to the sport enhancement issue is the value judgment that natural is good and artificial is bad: if an enhancement is judged natural, it is acceptable; if it is judged artificial, it is unacceptable. An additional problem is that this evaluative reasoning is not applied consistently.

Over time, many "enhancements" have become considered "normal" and even natural. Examples include the Fosbury Flop in 1968 in high jumping, which uses the whole body as an enhancement device, and the klapskate in 1997 in speed skating, which has a hinged blade (van Hilvoorde, Vos, and de Wert 2007). When first introduced, both generated significant controversy, being judged unnatural and unfair. On a more systemic note, early in the twentieth century it was not considered natural for women to compete in sports (Shogan 1999; Stebner and Trothen 2002). Today, each of these innovations is seen as natural in sport.

Hypobaric chambers and blood doping raise additional problems in that the physiological advantages they offer are produced by "natural substances." Hypobaric chambers are usually deemed acceptable as a training mechanism for high-altitude sports, even though a fairness or justice argument could be applied since this equipment is not universally accessible. Blood doping is seen as an unacceptable enhancement often on the grounds that it is unnatural.

Most problematic, the epistemological constructs of "normal" and "natural" have implications for who count as acceptable athletes. These constructs are informed by normative values. The case of genetic anomalies – sometimes called by the even more value-laden term "mutations" – illustrates the problem. As these "natural" advantages are made more visible by science, only some are assessed as excessive and therefore abnormal (bad); most are considered the product of good fortune – an enhanced normal (good). These assessments demonstrate that there is a fine line, heavily value-laden, between disability and extraordinary talent (van Hilvoorde and Landeweerd 2008). For example, Finnish athlete Eero Mantyranla, in the 1964 Winter Olympics, won two gold medals in cross-country skiing due in part to a rare mutation in the gene coding for his EPO receptor that resulted in a 25-50 percent increase in the oxygen-carrying capacity of his red blood cells (Aschwanden 2000; McCrory 2003). Olympic swimmer Michael Phelps has several advantageous genetic anomalies, including a wide wingspan, significant flexibility, and disproportionately large hands and feet (Dvorsky 2008).

The most widely known recent examples of elite athletes who do not appear to fit normative embodiment categories due to anomalies with which they were born are Semenya and Pistorius. Both have generated controversy and concern that they have unfair advantages over other runners. Yet Phelps's and Mantyranla's advantages have been seen as natural and therefore acceptable. In Semenya's case, natural was considered a bad thing because the possibility that she was intersexed, transgressing gender and sex categories, appeared to give her too much of an advantage; she was too much like a man to be a woman (Krane 2012; Jönsson 2007). Semenya's bodily appearance and record-breaking times visibly challenged constructed normative embodiment expectations and categories, including those of gender and sexuality. The question must be asked: why are Phelps's genetic anomalies considered good and Semenya's bad?

How one decides what constitutes a genetic "anomaly" is problematic. How one decides which anomalies are lucky and which are unacceptable and even somehow "unnatural" is more so. One must consider why the klapskate is seen as more natural than a possibly intersexed competitor or – potentially – than an athlete who opts for genetic modification technologies.

Although there are some exceptions,[6] in most cases, distinctions between natural and artificial presuppose that natural is morally superior and that it exists in an essential and discernable form. These distinctions are usually built on an essentialist understanding of normal as the dividing point, reinforcing judgments regarding who is a valid and valuable human being (Wolbring 2007; van Hilvoorde and Landeweerd 2008; Trothen 2011).

Individual Choice

Choice is not a simple criterion in the enhancement debate. Proponents of individual choice argue that athletes should be free to choose enhancements as long as they are medically safe and other athletes have the same freedom of choice (Miah 2004, 2005; Tamburrini 2007). Detractors argue that elite athletes do not have sufficient freedom to choose (Simon 2001, 2004; Loland 2002; Loland and Hoppeler 2012), pointing to cases such as the Tour de France, where the pressure to take enhancing substances mitigates consent. As Loland and Hoppeler (2012, 352) suggest, the multiplicity of political, economic, and social interests that can be applied to athletes makes choice a very complicated issue: "In the current situation the liberal approach is sociologically naïve and puts athletes at risk of exploitation." These issues were brought into the spotlight even more by the 2012 finding that Lance Armstrong had taken several performance-enhancing drugs, invalidating his seven Tour de France wins. Counter-responses to the argument that consent cannot truly be given by athletes cite paternalism, arguing that these athletes are capable of saying "no" even under pressure. This circular argument makes resolution unlikely.

Interestingly, even Miah (2004), who may well be the most extreme proponent of individual choice, argues that the choice should be consistent with an individual athlete's authentic humanity, not made for the purpose of gaining a covert competitive edge, but he tends to reduce the concept of choice to an extreme individualism. Most problematic, his argument assumes access to one's authentic self. Relational theorists have discovered that people do not "typically discover their own values by introspection ... [Rather,] persons *determine* their values through dialogue with others and action ... [Thus] we should not focus on the question 'what does a person want to do now?' but rather on 'what are the processes by which he/she has come to hold his current preferences?'" (Sherwin 2007, 177). In elite sport there is significant pressure to accept winning as the most important and sometimes the only value. Yet the questions of why and how winning has come to be the ultimate value are not often posed.

The high value placed on winning can divert attention away from the underlying messages regarding embodiment. For example, to win, one must fit into embodiment categories and classifications that are acceptable to elite sport. One's identity is assessed according to normative categories, including male or female, disabled or abled, and in some sports such as boxing, large or small. As is made clear elsewhere in this volume, identity formation is connected to how and what we know and value. Corporeal alteration(s) may enhance one's authenticity if the values and sociological dynamics underlying what we know are identified and critically examined.

Autonomy is a very important principle and cannot be reduced to the freedom to make individual choices. Autonomy must be considered in the context of systemic power distribution and the social reinforcement of normative values (see also Jakobsen, Chapter 1, and Holtmann, Chapter 6, this volume).[7] The issue of consent to added enhancements or tests to reveal by-chance advantages is much more complex than a simple notion of "yes" or "no." Not only does the pressure to win mitigate the ability to choose, but also operative are societal values and a deep-seated reward-punishment dynamic that inculcates the internalization and even propagation of these values. If Semenya had refused to be tested or to subscribe to whatever requirements may have been declared, she would not have been permitted to compete. She also faced global pressure through the media to "fit in" (Vannini and Fornssler 2010; Ratele 2011).

An approach focused only on individual choice also ignores distributive justice issues: there are many athletes who do not have the resources to access the techno-science even if it is available (Lebacqz 1997; Cahill 2001).

Fairness

Often, fairness is assumed to require a high degree of sameness. Extreme proponents of this approach see the minimizing of differences through enhancement technologies as desirable (Tamburrini 2007). For example, by increasing the oxygen-carrying capacity of red blood cells, the emerging gene therapy tentatively under the tradename of Repoxygen could minimize differences in athletes' endurance, thus levelling the playing field. In this line of reasoning, substances such as EPO could also be used to minimize difference and make competition fairer. As science creates additional technologies and pharmaceuticals, other differences could be detected and then "evened out" by providing correctives to the athletes who are at a disadvantage. Less extreme proponents want to minimize differences that are considered *unfair* advantages. Whether differences are evaluated as suspect rather than desirable or as unfair rather than simply lucky is related to what is valued.

In the Paralympics, fair competition assumes embodiment diversity and the recognition of this diversity in the structure of sporting events. For example, unlike the Olympics, in 2008 the Paralympics had "thirteen distinct finals for the men's one-hundred-meter dash, twelve for the women" (Murray 2010, 13). These categories are based on disability and severity. For example, one category is for track athletes with severe limb loss, and another is for swimmers with moderate visual impairment. Although this greater use of multiple categories is responsive to diversity in embodiment, a difficulty is the "'ongoing struggle' to find the right balance between a good competition based on differences in talent on the one hand and the demonstration of excellence within a group with relevant similar skills on the other" (van Hilvoorde and Landeweerd 2008, 99; see also Loland and Hoppeler 2012).

Sport categories are designed to address relevant embodiment differences so as to facilitate the best competition. However, there are many problems with the identification of significant and relevant embodiment differences. For example, although in track competitions there is an argument for a significant and relevant difference between men and women – insofar as people can and should be classified into these two narrowing, constructed groups (Shogan 1999) – there really is no good reason for this division in archery, yet it persists (Loland and Hoppeler 2012). Also consider that height is not a recognized difference in basketball competition, whereas size categories exist in boxing. The latter makes sense, but the former is arguably a notable oversight. It is interesting that in systemically less valued contexts, including the Paralympics, diversity and multiple embodiment categories are more likely to be expected and accepted. On the other hand, some argue that there should be no categories at the highest level of competition: the best athlete should win irrespective of embodiment particularities (Jönsson 2007). This "no category" approach eliminates problematic, value-laden embodiment categories but runs the risk of also eliminating the highest level of competition among a group of athletes who *generally* share many physical characteristics that are determined to be directly relevant to the performance of the particular sport. For example, largely because of their *generally* lesser physical strength and size compared to men, women rarely would achieve a place in hockey. But by eliminating women from hockey, we would also miss out on a different style of hockey (a bit slower so often more strategic, for example) played at the highest level.

Pistorius's very visible "Cheetah legs" have generated concern that they give him an unfair advantage (Burkett, McNamee, and Potthast 2011). Biomechanical testing and studies (e.g., Sutcliffe 2008; van Hilvoorde and Landeweerd 2008; Jones and Wilson 2009) led to Pistorius's successful appeal of his ban from IAAF competitions, allowing him to compete in the 2012 London Olympics, although he did not win. Pistorius was not the first disabled athlete to compete in the Olympic Games. However, in almost all of the other cases, there was no concern that the disability gave the person advantages over the other competitors.[8] Similarly, Semenya was allowed to compete after being judged to qualify as a woman. Again, the reasons for identifying some differences as unfair and others as simply fortunate and admirable (e.g., a basketball player's exceptional height) are problematic. In both cases, instead of recreating or reimagining embodiment categories, Semenya's differentness was managed or tolerated, and she was absorbed into the normative sex/gender category of woman.[9] Jönsson (2007, 241) summarizes the problematics of sex/gender categorization, arguing "that the rough distinctions we use to define people in terms of sex/gender tend to create and recreate sex/gender boundaries, and that this is the foundation of sex/gender-based discrimination in sport." The problem, Jönsson argues, is not the bodies that do not fit the categories but the categories themselves. Pistorius was found to have no net advantage from his prostheses and so was permitted to compete in the Olympics as an exception.

An acceptance of fairness as minimizing difference has implications not only for particular athletes such as Semenya and Pistorius but also more generally for elite sport and society. Proponents of this understanding of fairness argue for the use of emerging techno-science to "correct" embodiment differences between athletes. Enhancement technologies to even the playing field would likely become prolific: sport would become more of a performance of "competing bodies" and less a "test of persons" (Simon 2004, 13). Some argue that widening the gap between elite athletes and everyone else is desirable because it increases entertainment, which is what people want when they watch sport (Tamburrini 2007). Others disagree, pointing to the identification of spectators with the athletes and particularly the desire of spectators to believe that effort, not simply luck or technology, plays a meaningful role in determining the outcome of sports competition (Caplan 2008).

Even if techno-science enhancements are not embraced as the solution to embodiment diversity, this diversity will become more visible, and this increased visibility will make it harder to maintain what I call sport's "meritocracy illusion." This term refers to the conviction that anyone, given sufficient training, dedication, and heart, can become a star athlete. If followers and fans identify with the athletes and dream of achieving the fastest time or lifting the most weight, a widened gap will damage this dream or will inspire people to use techno-science enhancements themselves. Not only will the belief that elite athletes are just like us be dissolved, but more important, so too will the hope for athletic success that presupposes a significant degree of embodiment sameness. In Canada perhaps the most common example of this is the belief that any male child can "make" the National Hockey League. Countless parents invest their resources in this hope, inflicting damage on themselves and their aspiring children (Gillis 2013). The increasing visibility of embodiment diversity indicates what has been known at some level for a long time: some people are physically advantaged and some disadvantaged at particular sports. Yet the idea that anyone can succeed given enough effort (Caplan 2008; Nowotny and Testa 2010; Loland 2012) persists as both a conviction and a hope. In the religion of elite sport, understandings of embodiment diversity and the construction of hope are connected; hope thus far in this religion has been built on the presupposition and prizing of embodiment sameness. The persistence of this belief in significant sameness could end up serving as a rationale for the use of techno-science enhancements to sustain this conviction, particularly as the diversity of bodies is made more visible.

The revelation that Lance Armstrong took enhancing substances and lied about it devastated fans who could no longer believe that it was possible for a cancer survivor to come back and win seven Tour de France competitions without using prohibited enhancement substances. Similarly, but more extreme, was Pistorius's fall from the moral high ground when he was arrested for the murder of girlfriend Reeva Steenkamp. In South Africa the media reported that he was regarded as "a hero by both blacks and whites, transcending the racial divide of the country" (Wire Services 2013). The most admired sports heroes are those who most clearly personify the rags to riches story; to them are attributed moral ideals and fortitude. These success stories involve the hero overcoming barrier(s) and eventually winning in competition while maintaining exemplary conformity to societal and sport rules.

Popular sources of the hope and meaning attached to elite sport must be reimagined. Without such reimagining, the temptation to make the "meritocracy illusion" real will be a strong influence on arguments for the unrestricted use of enhancements. I surmise that the desire to maintain this illusion and the hope constructed upon the presumption of sameness is often behind the argument that enhancement technologies should be used to create a more level playing field. To use a Judeo-Christian metaphor, we want to return to the Garden, but the Garden is not there as we have imagined it. And as Nowotny and Testa (2010, 20) observe, "The more that equality turns out to be a fiction, the more it seems necessary to cling to it." The flattening of differences will not add meaning to sports competition; such competition is built on human diversity. This is the paradox.

Internal Goods of (the) Sport

Some contend that the issue of techno-science and enhancement in sport is really about the meaning of sport, and they propose reframing the issue in terms of the goods of each sport and sometimes the goods of sport more generally. A concern is whether enhancement technologies will render meaningless the defining tests of each sport and thus the sport as well. For example, super swimsuits were banned partly on the basis that they distort the nature of the sport of swimming; the basic test of one's ability to manoeuvre through water was made too easy by polyurethane suits, making it impossible to compare these newer times with past win times (Burkett, McNamee, and Potthast 2011). Similarly, some object to Pistorius's participation in the Olympics on the basis that he is not running but is "showing another and extra skill, namely handling his prosthesis in an extremely talented way" (van Hilvoorde and Landeweerd 2010, 2226; see also Edwards 2008). However, measurable criteria for determining what defines running are vague and can thus be used to justify arguments of inclusion or exclusion (Jones and Wilson 2009).

Gleaves (2010) takes an internal-goods approach a step further, arguing that for a sport to remain meaningful, its defining tests must demonstrate three characteristics: suitability, durability, and continuity. He gives the example of baseball in America; this sport, he surmises, is so much more successful in the United States than in the United Kingdom because of the American values it exemplifies: both "individual agency [i.e., a lone batter against a single pitcher] as well as cooperative agency [e.g., the team advancing of runners and sacrifice plays]" (ibid., 279). Enhancements that might change the suitability of the tests of baseball to the American culture would likely render it less popular. For example, if techno-science could enable hitters to achieve homeruns much more often, the teamwork necessary to baseball winning would not be so important, thus making it less attractive to an American culture that is still interested in something beyond the individual.

This approach to the enhancement issue assumes that "successful" sport fits into existing socio-cultural norms and values and that this fit is a good thing. However, fitting in, attracting viewership, and generating financial gain do not necessarily serve the overall social good but reproduce normative ideals and values. Sport can be a location where diversity flourishes and where those who do not "fit" are built up. The question arises of whether this attentiveness to diversity and inclusion is more appropriate to less competitive sport.[10]

This is a difficult question whose answer depends in part on how one sees the internal goods of elite sport. Competition is important, and arguably the best competition occurs when the best competitors are matched against each other. If elite sport is regarded as the pinnacle of sport, then having a different set of goods attached to this level sends a conflicted message to sport participants and followers. The values espoused in elite sport remain the ideal and the hope. If embodiment diversity is recognized and valued as the underpinning of competitive sport, the goal will not be the creation of a (more) level playing field to further the illusion of a normative sameness. Rather, more marginalized values such as diversity, inclusion, and the playing of the game might be regarded as sport's internal goods. Although this shift seems to be happening at less visible levels, it remains strongly contested in elite sport. Similarly, whereas invisible embodiment differences are often acceptable, visible embodiment differences are often contested. As Nowotny and Testa (2010, 25) explain, "Oscar Pistorius is punished for the visibility of his prostheses because he publicly displays his difference from his normal competitors ... It is thought-provoking that a society proud of its ideal of equality sees a threat to sports precisely when technology enables a handicapped person to overtake his nonhandicapped competitors." Further, that Pistorius wanted to compete in the "normal" Olympics underlies the status differential between the Paralympics and Olympics (Swartz and Watermeyer 2008). The inclusion of some non-normative appearing bodies in the normative Olympics is not an effective means of altering normative values or restrictive normalizing categories. Elite sport is the location of not only reproduced but also amplified global normative values and ideals associated with physical appearance, sexuality, gender, winning, and efficiency.

What These Approaches Tell Us: Values, Ideals, and Hope

As a secular religion that defies the separation of the spirit from the body and the sacred from the profane, sport has transformative qualities and potential. In sport, the body is the locus of spirituality. This disrupts the binary construction of the sacred and the profane. And it fosters both the valuing of embodiment and, potentially, a diversity of embodiment that embraces those who are not only extraordinarily fit but also anomalous. Yet not all such bodies are valued similarly. This diversity is tolerated and even admired but only until normative embodiment categories are disrupted by very visible differences.

Replicating normative technological and social values, the enhancement debate in elite sport is shaped by ideals of naturalness, normality, meritocracy, and success. The meaning of these ideals is influenced by several values, including winning, efficiency, status, money, and conformity (or fitting in). Each of the four main approaches to the enhancement issue – the artificial-natural distinction, individual choice, fairness, and internal goods – does not critically investigate these underlying ideals and normative values but instead tends to accept them.

The implications of this acceptance include the replication and amplification of these values as they affect approaches to embodiment diversity. Particularly as science makes clearer the fallacy of universal claims about embodiment and creates more options for tailoring or recreating bodies, these values become increasingly important. Techno-science is adding to embodiment diversity and, in so doing, is making it increasingly difficult to maintain normative embodiment categories. It is not difficult to imagine increasingly posthuman athletes who blur the distinction between human and machine. "Cheetah legs" will become normal, as will athletes whose bodies defy gender categorization. Technology brings a value set; we shape our tools and our tools shape us. Similarly, as a secular religion, sport both manifests and challenges normative culture and values (Overman 1997; Trothen 2006). Elite sport values winning most highly. As it stands, bodies that win and accommodate normative conceptions of appearance – including epistemological embodiment constructs based on male-female and abled-disabled binaries – are accepted and prized in elite sport. However, these normative conceptions are being challenged, particularly by techno-science innovations.

Athletes are pushed to conform visibly to these often contradictory or paradoxical values. For example, Lance Armstrong was expected both to continue winning the Tour de France and to be natural, refraining from the use of banned substances. Caster Semenya was expected both to prove herself "glamorous" and feminine and to be powerful and strong enough to win (Ratele 2011). Similarly, highly "successful" disabled athletes will continue to strive to "graduate" to competition in the "normal" Olympics.

The visibility of diverse bodies is necessary to show that normative embodiment categories and their entwined gender and sexual implications – including the construction of abled-disabled, female-male, and gay-straight dichotomies[11] – do not work for all bodies. As King (2008, 431) posits, visibility or "outing" is necessary and important in that it "allows subjects to be seen and often to speak but ... does not lead automatically to the erasure of stereotypes, the end of violence, the redistribution of resources, or to greater freedom." The intersection of techno-science with elite sport's high level of competitiveness has contributed to the visibility and development of embodiment diversity. However, something more than greater visibility is needed if we are to go from destabilizing these normative epistemologies and values to undertaking a reconstruction (DeMarrais, Castillo, and Earle 1996).

This something more may be the erosion of a normatively (and falsely) constructed hope in this very popular secular religion. As normative categories of epistemological embodiment are challenged by nonconforming bodies, so too is the hope that has been located in the ideal of meritocracy (sameness). Coupled with the possibilities offered by techno-science, the faith claim that we alone can create whatever we truly desire (and that we can easily know what we truly desire) could result in a narrowing of who is acceptable. However, there is also the possibility that the growing visibility of embodiment diversity could provide an opportunity to intentionally explore values and ideals by asking what provides meaning and hope. In short, what do we want to enhance and how can we best do this enhancing? The location of what Jakobsen (Chapter 1, this volume) terms "moral panic" or "moral preoccupation" is very relevant to the topic of elite sport and enhancement. The panic generated by visibly different Olympic athletes is not only a reaction to the disruption of embodiment categories but also, at a deeper level, a reaction to this crisis of hope.

The sport enhancement debate has been defined as the question of where to draw the line between acceptable and unacceptable advantages. This debate, as we have seen, is informed by underlying and usually unexamined values and hopes pertaining to embodiment diversity. Techno-science enhancement innovations will add to visible embodiment diversity. In so doing, they will make it increasingly difficult to identify who has what sexual preferences and desires and what people's sexual practices might be. No doubt, this ambiguity will generate more anxiety, as it will become that much more difficult to categorize and control sexualities and their expressions.

In sum, the debate over enhancement is a debate over embodiment diversity and values. As science presents more possibilities for self-enhancement, questions about values will become even more pressing. Are normative values that reinforce established embodiment categories sufficient or desirable? I suggest that there is great value in diversity and that sport as a secular religion is built on presumptions of bodily goodness and diversity. Sport, as a secular religion, could more deliberately cultivate its own set of values, one that does not simply conform to normative constructs and ways of knowing. By fostering an appreciation and delight in embodiment diversity, sport could become a secular religion that cultivates hope centred on an embodiment diversity.

Approaches to the enhancement debate reflect the inadequacies of normative views of embodiment. Embodied humans defy neat static categories. Sport, as a widespread secular religion, is an important social force in the propagation of values regarding embodiment diversity. Both the significance of the enhancement debate to the "meritocracy illusion" and the tenacity of this illusion (as a source of hope) suggest that conformity to normative values concerning embodiment is part of sport's religious dimension but not necessarily the whole story. As diversity is made more visible by techno-science, hope must either shift its locus or die. As a religion, sport offers the transformative possibility that hope and meaning can be relocated in the very thing that is resisted: the beauty of diverse bodies.

As this chapter only begins to explore the topic of sport, enhancement, religion, and embodiment, the following are some further questions for reflection and discussion:

- What might be some implications of this discussion of embodiment categories in sport?
- Where might elite sport go with the enhancement question?
- How might amateur sport differ from elite sport in relation to embodiment diversity?
- Where might hope become located in the secular religion of sport?
- What does it mean to enhance oneself? In the quest to become "better," how do we know or can we know what makes humanity "better"?
- Are there or should there be limits to the use of techno-science to change being human?
- What values should inform decisions about enhancement options in sport?

Many athletes have experiences that they understand as religious or spiritual (Sanford 2007). As philosopher of religion Michael Novak (1993, 162) insists, "To have a religion, you need to have a way to exhilarate the human body, and desire, and will, and the sense of beauty, and a sense of oneness with the universe and other humans." At its best, sport does this. Normative values and ideals are being both challenged and replicated in the sport enhancement debate. Athletes and sport followers are pushing restrictive notions of both religion and embodiment. It may be that humanity is approaching a turning point.

Notes

This chapter was made possible through the Lilly Theological Research Grants Program.

1 In keeping with these theorists (and similar to Nason-Clark, Chapter 9, this volume), I understand embodiment as inextricably tied to sexuality. It should be noted that a number of contemporary theologians have drawn similar links centred on interpretations of Christianity's incarnational focus, including James B. Nelson (1996, 214), who understands sexuality as "present in all of human experience." Theological ethicist Marvin M. Ellison (1996, 222) refers to sexuality as "our embodied sensuous connectedness to all reality [and] ... our human capacity and longing for intimacy and communion."
2 Horn et al (2005) have borrowed the term "body-selves" from Nelson (1978, 40).
3 Contemporary studies support the notion that gender is "an identity tenuously constituted in time – an identity instituted through a stylized repetition of acts" (Butler 2003, 415).
4 An exploration of the binary construction of the spiritual and the religious is outside of the scope of this chapter but has been addressed by others (e.g., Lebacqz and Driskill 2000; Rose 2001).
5 This would not have been the first time that a male-appearing competitor had identified as a "woman" at the elite sport level. Runner Stella Walsh won gold in the 1932 Olympics and was discovered in 1980, through an autopsy, to have been male, generating debate about whether cheating had occurred or whether the problem was more with the restrictive sex/gender categories (Jönsson 2007).
6 Perhaps most notably, Loland and Hoppeler (2012) propose using the concept of human phenotypic plasticity to evaluate enhancements. Training, they argue, should use the body's particular phenotypic plasticity, which is a combination of genetic and environmental factors, and any substance that ignores it by bypassing the body's physiological reaction patterns (e.g., by taking "short cuts" to get the desired effect, such as EPO) should be prohibited. Although this approach understands that each body has its own normality, it does not address the issues of germ-line genetic modification technologies, technological additions, or the failure of embodiment categories to be inclusive. However, Loland and Hoppeler note that their model does not address all enhancement cases.
7 Feminist theorists such as Susan Sherwin (2007) posit a "relational autonomy," underscoring the communal and contextual nature of this principle.
8 An athlete with a wooden leg, George Eyser, won three gold medals in gymnastics at the 1904 Olympics. Blind runner Marla Runyan competed in the 1,500 metre race in the 2000 Olympics and finished in eighth place. More controversially, Neroli Fairhall competed in archery in the 1984 Olympics while in a wheelchair, which some argued gave him an advantage (van Hilvoorde and Landeweerd 2008; Burkett, McNamee, and Potthast 2011).

9 As Ratele (2011) notes, the concepts of sex and gender are conflated, pointing to the fact that both, at least in part, are constructs.
10 Studies have suggested that nonelite but competitive sport communities and participation are contexts for the cultivation of alternative values. For example, after identifying the dynamic of social control as operative for many gay, male marathoners, sports sociologists William Bridel and Geneviève Rail (2007, 131, 139) conclude that although social norms influenced in some ways a group of distance runners, these runners prioritized the more marginalized value of "personal achievement" over winning and created an alternative construction of physical attractiveness. This transformative potential of sport was also evidenced in a later qualitative study by Ravel and Rail (2008) of fourteen young francophone sportswomen from Montreal. Building on previous studies that showed sport providing "a refuge for many women with nonconventional sexualities" (ibid., 5), the researchers found that "sport was generally constructed by the participants as providing support to gaie athletes" and as "resisting heteronormativity" (ibid., 17, 18). Communities based on the body as a locus of power and strength can foster both communal and individual transformations regarding sexualities and embodiment (Sanford 2007, 888-91).
11 Attached to these dichotomous categories are assumptions that further devalue and disempower the negated category. For example, the disabled body tends to be desexed, as are elderly and cognitively disabled bodies (Stuart 2000).

References

Albanese, C. 1982. *America: Religions and Religion*. Belmont, CA: Wadsworth.

Aschwanden, C. 2000. Gene Cheats. *New Scientist*, 15 January, 24-29.

–. 2012. The Future of Cheating in Sports. *Smithsonian Magazine*, July. http://www.smithsonianmag.com/science-nature/The-Future-of-Cheating-in-Sports-160285295.html.

Austin, M.W. 2010. Sports as Exercises in Spiritual Formation. *Journal of Spiritual Formation and Soul Care* 3 (1): 66-78.

Bain-Selbo, E. 2009. *Game Day and God: Football, Faith, and Politics in the American South*. Macon, GA: Mercer University Press.

Bellah, R.N. 1967. Civil Religion in America. In *Religion in America*, ed. W.G. McLoughlin and R.N. Bellah, 3-23. Boston: Houghton Mifflin.

Bouchard, C. 2012. Genetics and Sports Performance. Paper presented at the International Convention on Science, Education and Medicine in Sport, Glasgow, United Kingdom, 20 July.

Bridel, W., and G. Rail. 2007. Sport, Sexuality, and the Production of (Resistant) Bodies: De-/Re-Constructing the Meanings of Gay Male Marathon Corporeality. *Sociology of Sport Journal* 24 (2): 127-44.

Burkett, B., M. McNamee, and W. Potthast. 2011. Shifting Boundaries in Sports Technology and Disability: Equal Rights or Unfair Advantage in the Case of Oscar Pistorius? *Disability and Society* 26 (5): 643-54.

Butler, J. 1990. *Gender Trouble: Feminism and the Subversion of Identity*. New York and London: Routledge.

–. 2003. Performative Acts and Gender Constitution: An Essay in Phenomenology and Feminist Theory. In *Feminist Theory Reader: Local and Global Perspectives*, ed. C.R. McCann and S-K. Kim, 419-30. New York: Routledge.

Cahill, L.S. 2001. Cloning and Sin: A Neibuhrian Analysis and a Catholic, Liberationist Response. In *Beyond Cloning: Religion and the Remaking of Humanity*, ed. R. Cole-Turner, 97-110. Harrisburg, PA: Trinity Press International.

Callaway, K. 2013. *Scoring Transcendence: Contemporary Film Music as Religious Experience*. Waco, TX: Baylor University Press.

Caplan, A.L. 2008. Does the Biomedical Revolution Spell the End of Sport? *British Journal of Sports Medicine* 42 (12): 996-97.

Davey, A. 2002. *Urban Christianity and Global Order: Theological Resources for an Urban Future*. Peabody, MA: Hendrickson.

Davies, G.A. 2011. London 2012 Olympics: Double Amputee Oscar Pistorius Makes 400m Qualifying Time. *Telegraph* (London), 24 March. http://www.telegraph.co.uk/sport/othersports/olympics/8403343/London-2012-Olympics-double-amputee-Oscar-Pistorius-makes-400m-qualifying-time.html.

DeMarrais, E., L.J. Castillo, and T. Earle. 1996. Ideology, Materialization, and Power Strategies. *Current Anthropology* 37 (1): 15-31.

Dickey Young, P. 2002. The Resurrection of the Body? A Feminist Look at the Question of Transcendence. *Feminist Theology* 10 (30): 44-51.

Dvorsky, G. 2008. Michael Phelps: "Naturally" Transhuman. 19 August. http://ieet.org/index.php/IEET/print/2575.

Edwards, L., and C. Jones. 2009. Postmodernism, Queer Theory and Moral Judgment in Sport. *International Review for the Sociology of Sport* 44 (4): 331-44.

Edwards, S.D. 2008. "Should Oscar Pistorius be Excluded from the 2008 Olympic Games?" *Sport Ethics and Philosophy* 2 (2): 112-25.

Ellison, M.M. 1996. Sexuality and Spirituality: An Intimate – and Intimidating – Connection. In *Christian Perspectives on Gender and Sexuality*, ed. E. Stuart and A. Thatcher, 220-27. Grand Rapids, MI: William B. Eerdmans.

Fagg, L.W. 2003. Are There Intimations of Divine Transcendence in the Physical World? *Zygon* 38 (3): 559-72.

Foucault, M. 1979. *Discipline and Punish: The Birth of the Prison*. New York: Vintage.

–. 1988. *Technologies of the Self: A Seminar with Michel Foucault*. Ed. L.H. Martin, H. Gutman, and P.H. Hutton. Boston: University of Massachusetts Press.

Friedmann, T. 2012. Genetics and Sports Performance. Paper presented at the International Convention on Science, Education and Medicine in Sport, Glasgow, United Kingdom, 20 July.

Gebara, I. 2002. *Out of the Depths: Women's Experience of Evil and Salvation*. Minneapolis, MN: Fortress.

Gillis, C. 2013. The Real Scandal in Hockey: Ken Campbell on the Problem with Canada's Obsession. *Maclean's*, 20 January. http://www2.macleans.ca/2013/01/20/year-round-training-and-320000-wont-guarantee-an-nhl-career-or-even-a-future-fan.

Gleaves, J. 2010. No Harm, No Foul? Justifying Bans of Safe Performance-Enhancing Drugs. *Sport, Ethics and Philosophy* 4 (3): 270-83.

Habermas, J. 1968. *Knowledge and Human Interests*. Boston: Beacon.

Horn, M.J., R.L. Piedmont, G.M. Fialkowski, R.J. Wicks, and M.E. Hunt. 2005. Sexuality and Spirituality: The Embodied Spirituality Scale. *Theology and Sexuality* 12 (1): 81-102.

Isherwood, L., ed. 2000. *The Good News of the Body: Sexual Theology and Feminism*. New York: New York University Press.

Jackson, S., and M. Csikszentmihalyi. 1999. *Flow in Sports: The Keys to Optimal Experiences and Performance*. Champaign, IL: Human Kinetics.

Jones, C., and C. Wilson. 2009. Defining Advantage and Athletic Performance: The Case of Oscar Pistorius. *European Journal of Sport Science* 9 (2): 125-31.

Jönsson, K. 2007. Who's Afraid of Stella Walsh? On Gender, "Gene Cheaters," and the Promises of Cyborg Athletes. *Sport, Ethics and Philosophy* 1 (2): 239-62.

Kahane, G. 2011. Mastery without Mystery: Why There Is No Promethean Sin in Enhancement. *Journal of Applied Philosophy* 28 (4): 355-68.

Kelly, P. 2011. Flow, Sport and the Spiritual Life. In *Theology, Ethics and Transcendence in Sports*, ed. J. Parry, M. Nesti, and N. Watson, 163-77. London: Routledge.

King, S. 2008. What's Queer about (Queer) Sport Sociology Now? A Review Essay. *Sociology of Sport Journal* 25 (4): 419-42.

Krane, V. 2012. Gender, Identity and Ethics. Paper presented at the International Convention on Science, Education and Medicine in Sport, Glasgow, United Kingdom, 21 July.

Ladd, T., and J.A. Mathisen. 1999. *Muscular Christianity: Evangelical Protestants and the Development of American Sport*. Grand Rapids, MI: Baker Books.

Lebacqz, K. 1997. Genes, Justice and Clones. In *Human Cloning: Religious Responses*, ed. R. Cole-Turner, 49-57. Louisville, KY: Westminster John Knox Press.

Lebacqz, K., and J.D. Driskill. 2000. *Ethics and Spiritual Care: A Guide for Pastors, Chaplains and Spiritual Directors*. Nashville, TN: Abingdon.

Legge, M.J. 2006. Social Ethics, Women, and Religion. In *The Encyclopedia of Women and Religion in North America*, ed. R.S. Keller and R. Radford Ruether, vol. 1, 52-62. Indianapolis: Indiana University Press.

Loland, S. 2002. *Fair Play in Sport: A Moral Norm System*. London: Routledge.
–. 2012. A Well Balanced Life Based on "The Joy of Effort": Olympic Hype or a Meaningful Ideal? *Sport, Ethics and Philosophy* 6 (2): 155-65.
Loland, S., and H. Hoppeler. 2012. Justifying Anti-Doping: The Fair Opportunity Principle and the Biology of Performance Enhancement. *European Journal of Sport Science* 12 (4): 347-53.
Lynch, G. 2007. What Is This "Religion" in the Study of Religion and Popular Culture? In *Between Sacred and Profane: Researching Religion and Popular Culture*, ed. G. Lynch, 125-42. London: I.B. Tauris.
Macur, J. 2007. Rule Jostles Runners Who Race to Their Own Tune. *New York Times*, 1 November.
Marcuse, H. 1964. *One-Dimensional Man: Studies in the Ideology of Advanced Industrial Society*. Boston: Beacon.
Martinkova, I., and J. Parry. 2011. Zen, Movement and Sports. In *Theology, Ethics and Transcendence in Sports*, ed. J. Parry, M. Nesti, and N. Watson, 211-22. London: Routledge.
Mathisen, J. 2001. American Sport as Folk Religion: Examining a Test of Its Strength. In *From Season to Season: Sport as American Religion*, ed. J.L. Price, 141-62. Macon, GA: Mercer University Press.
McCrory, P. 2003. Super Athletes or Gene Cheats? *British Journal of Sports Medicine* 37 (3): 192-93.
Miah, A. 2004. *Genetically Modified Athletes: Biomedical Ethics, Gene Doping, and Sport*. New York: Routledge.
–. 2005. From Anti-Doping to a "Performance Policy" Sport Technology, Being Human, and Doing Ethics. *European Journal of Sport Science* 5 (1): 51-57.
Moltmann, J. 1985. *God in Creation: A New Theology of Creation and the Spirit of God*. Trans. M. Kohl. San Francisco: Harper and Row.
–. 1992. *The Spirit of Life: A Universal Affirmation*. Trans. M. Kohl. Minneapolis, MN: Fortress.
Murray, T.H. 2010. Making Sense of Fairness in Sports. *Hastings Center Report* 40 (2): 13-15.
Nelson, J.B. 1978. *Embodiment: An Approach to Sexuality and Christian Theology*. Minneapolis, MN: Augsburg.
–. 1996. Reuniting Sexuality and Spirituality. In *Christian Perspectives on Gender and Sexuality*, ed. E. Stuart and A. Thatcher, 213-19. Grand Rapids, MI: William B. Eerdmans.
Novak, M. 1993. The Joy of Sports. In *Religion and Sport: The Meeting of Sacred and Profane*, ed. C.S. Prebish, 151-72. Westport, CT: Greenwood.
Nowotny, H., and G. Testa. 2010. *Naked Genes: Reinventing the Human in the Molecular Age*. Trans. M. Cohen. Cambridge, MA: MIT Press.

Overman, S.J. 1997. *The Influence of the Protestant Ethic on Sport and Recreation.* Aldershot, UK: Ashgate.

Prebish, C.S., ed. 1993. *Religion and Sport: The Meeting of Sacred and Profane.* Westport, CT: Greenwood.

Price, J.L. 2001. From Sabbath Proscriptions to Super Sunday Celebrations: Sports and Religion in America. In *From Season to Season: Sport as American Religion,* ed. J.L. Price, 15-38. Macon, GA: Mercer University Press.

Ratele, K. 2011. Looks: Subjectivity as Commodity. *Agenda: Empowering Women for Gender Equity* 25 (4): 92-103.

Ravel, B., and G. Rail. 2008. From Straight to Gaie? Quebec Sportswomen's Discursive Constructions of Sexuality and Destabilizations of the Linear Coming Out Process. *Journal of Sport and Social Issues* 32 (1): 4-23.

Rose, S. 2001. Is the Term "Spirituality" a Word That Everyone Uses, But Nobody Knows What Anyone Means By It? *Journal of Contemporary Religion* 16 (2): 193-207.

Sanford, A.W. 2007. Pinned on Karma Rock: Whitewater Kayaking as Religious Experience. *Journal of the American Academy of Religion* 75 (4): 875-95.

Sherwin, S. 2007. Genetic Enhancement, Sports and Relational Autonomy. *Sport, Ethics and Philosophy* 1 (2): 171-80.

Shogan, D. 1999. *The Making of High-Performance Athletics: Discipline, Diversity, and Ethics.* Toronto: University of Toronto Press.

Simon, R.L. 2001. Good Competition and Drug-Enhanced Performance. In *Ethics in Sport,* ed. W.J. Morgan, K.V. Meier, and A.J. Schneider, 119-29. Champaign, IL: Human Kinetics, 2001.

–. 2004. *Fair Play: The Ethics of Sport.* 2nd ed. Boulder, CO: Westview.

Sinclair-Faulkner, T. 1977. A Puckish Reflection on Religion in Canada. In *Religion and Culture in Canada/Religion et Culture au Canada,* ed. P. Slater, 383-405. Ottawa: Corporation Canadienne des Sciences Religieuses/Canadian Corporation for Studies in Religion.

Stebner, E.J., and T.J. Trothen. 2002. A Diamond Is Forever? Women, Baseball and a Pitch for a Radically Inclusive Community. In *The Faith of 50 Million: Baseball, Religion, and American Culture,* ed. C.H. Evans and W.R. Herzog II, 167-86. Louisville, KY: Westminster John Knox Press.

Stuart, E. 2000. Disruptive Bodies: Disability, Embodiment and Sexuality. In *The Good News of The Body: Sexual Theology and Feminism,* ed. L. Isherwood, 166-84. New York: New York University Press.

Sutcliffe, M. 2008. Amputee Sprinter Treads Uneven Track. *Ottawa Citizen,* 13 January. http://www.canada.com/ottawacitizen/columnists/story.html?id=51d55c3d-72fd-4261-b138-35a0f1709b1f.

Swartz, L., and B. Watermeyer. 2008. Cyborg Anxiety: Oscar Pistorius and the Boundaries of What It Means to Be Human. *Disability and Society* 23 (2): 187-90.

Tamburrini, C.M. 2007. What's Wrong with Genetic Inequality? The Impact of Genetic Technology on Elite Sports and Society. *Sport, Ethics and Philosophy* 1 (2): 229-38.

Trothen, T.J. 2006. Hockey: A Divine Sport? Canada's National Sport in Relation to Embodiment, Community, and Hope. *Studies in Religion/Sciences Religieuses* 35 (2): 291-305.

–. 2009. The Sporting Spirit? Gene Doping, Bioethics, and Religion. *International Journal of Religion and Sport* 1: 1-20.

–. 2011. Better Than Normal? Constructing Genetically Modified Athletes and a Relational Theological Ethic. In *Theology, Ethics and Transcendence in Sports*, ed. J. Parry, M. Nesti, and N. Watson, 64-81. New York: Routledge.

–. 2012. The Technoscience Enhancement Debate in Sports: What's Religion Got to Do With It? In *Sports and Christianity: Historical and Contemporary Perspectives*, ed. N.J. Watson and A. Parker, 207-24. New York: Routledge.

van Hilvoorde, I., and L. Landeweerd. 2008. Disability or Extraordinary Talent: Francesco Lentini (Three Legs) versus Oscar Pistorius (No Legs). *Sports, Ethics and Philosophy* 2 (2): 97-111.

–. 2010. Enhancing Disabilities: Transhumanism Under the Veil of Inclusion. *Disability and Rehabilitation* 32 (26): 2222-27.

van Hilvoorde, I., R. Vos, and G. de Wert. 2007. Flopping, Klapping and Gene Doping: Dichotomies between "Natural" and "Artificial" in Elite Sport. *Social Studies of Science* 37 (2): 173-200.

Vannini, A., and B. Fornssler. 2010. Girl, Interrupted: Interpreting Semenya's Body, Gender Verification Testing, and Public Discourse. *Cultural Studies Critical Methodologies* 11 (3): 243-57.

Wire Services. 2013. Murder or Accident? *Kingston Whig-Standard*, 23 February, 18.

Wolbring, G. 2007. NBICS, Other Convergences, Ableism and the Culture of Peace. 15 April. http://www.innovationwatch-archive.com/choiceisyours/choiceisyours-2007-04-15.htm.

9

Strong Spirits, Abused Bodies
SOCIAL, POLITICAL, AND THEOLOGICAL REFLECTIONS

Nancy Nason-Clark

The journey toward justice, accountability, healing, and wholeness in the aftermath of domestic violence involves much uncharted territory, especially so when those impacted are highly committed religious people. Women who have been victimized by the men they love often hold out hope that, if only their abusers could be held accountable and receive intervention, the violence would stop. This is especially true of women of deep religious convictions (Nason-Clark and Clark Kroeger 2004). As a result, responders need to understand both the issue of domestic violence and the nature of religious faith. Insights and resources that harness both the language of the spirit and the language of contemporary culture are rare, a result of the delicate terrain for building bridges between secular and sacred sources of assistance. Building bridges of common language, perspective, respect, and understanding between sacred and secular sources of assistance presents both opportunities and challenges (Nason-Clark 2013).

For over twenty years, I have been conducting research among religious victims, survivors, and perpetrators of domestic violence and among the professionals who walk alongside them (Nason-Clark 2000, 2004, 2009). In this chapter, I attempt to tease apart some of the social, political, and theological underpinnings of abuse within communities of faith. Understanding the common features of women with strong spirits but abused bodies can help us to reduce the prevalence and persistence of abuse among co-religionists and support best practices for those who suffer. In part, the issues raised in the various chapters in this volume push us to consider anew what identity means in the context of the sexual and the religious. Heather Shipley and Andrew Kam-Tuck Yip highlight the constraints of framing religious identity as prescribing rigid or specific narratives, beliefs, or practices related to sexuality or even to the mention of sex in public discourse. As well, Pamela Dickey Young and Donald Boisvert vividly portray the level of discomfort that is experienced by religious organizations and their hierarchies when controversies regarding sexuality leave the private sphere and enter broader public discourse. In all of these examples, the boundaries are pushed and blurred: sometimes certain kinds of sexual relationships are marginalized, and sometimes certain forms of religious expression are discounted. In their chapters, too, Tracy Trothen and Catherine Holtmann challenge the notion that religion and sexuality operate only, or even primarily, within tightly constructed and guarded boundaries. To be sure, control is often an issue; in almost any narrative of a victim of violence, control is a key feature. But, as we will see, in the stories of survival, there are also hints of freedom, justice, choice, and agency – themes that also emerge in the fieldwork I have undertaken over the years.

In the interface of religion and domestic violence, issues involving sexuality are almost always lurking just beneath the surface, for any discussion of gender and violence is intertwined with notions of sex, with notions of sexuality and sexual expression, and with violence that is both physical and sexual. Throughout my fieldwork, women victims often used the general terms "abuse" or "domestic violence" to cover up the explicit and painful experiences and humiliations they had endured. One instance of such "abuse" is sexual name-calling, such as using terms like "slut" and "whore." For a highly religious woman who sees sexual purity as an important personal virtue, such name-calling is a poignant example of an abuser's desire to humiliate her strong spirit; it is a strategy of control aimed at denouncing and silencing the spiritual resources at her personal disposal.

Both the violence itself, including its many and varied manifestations, and the implications and impact of the violence may have sexual overtones. Just as sexuality is an embodied, lived experience, so too is violence for those who are its victims – and who live to become survivors. Although few have talked about it openly, strong spirits and abused bodies are often cohabiting – intermixed in the ongoing saga of family life when violence strikes at home.

My research for this chapter included surveys and interviews conducted with large samples of conservative Protestant clergy as well as mainline ministers. My other studies have included focus groups with church women, interviews with survivors, case file analyses of abusive men who have been participants in a batterer intervention program, as well as interviews and focus groups with men who act abusively. Some of my studies have considered the stories of those who walk alongside the victim or the perpetrator – from the perspective of either the criminal justice system or therapeutic agencies. Over the years, my research has included both qualitative and quantitative studies, and it is in the rich blending of various strategies that one can observe both the broader picture and its more detailed features.

Strong Spirits

Religious women are often very resilient when crisis impacts their lives.[1] In part, this is a reflection of the fact that they understand their congregation as a "church family" and look to others there for support and emotional assistance.[2] Within conservative religious circles, there is often a highly developed understanding of the life of faith and of those resources, both internal and external to the individual, that can be harnessed for strength in the face of obstacles. For women who are members of faith communities that value "separateness from the world," there is often a high expectation to serve others in their faith community during times of need and a strong familiarity with, and warmth toward, their "sisters" in the fold. When crisis in the family occurs, it is not uncommon for many of these women to look first and foremost to other women within their religious tradition for help. In fact, I have argued (Nason-Clark 1997; Kroeger and Nason-Clark 2010) that one of the best kept secrets of congregational life is the strong support women offer to each other under the umbrella of their faith community: it is often not recognized by men co-religionists, and it frequently occurs under the radar screen of pastors and other religious leaders. It is what women do to support each other – in good times and when times are anything but good. Ask almost any analyst of contemporary patterns in Christianity's church life about the difference that gender makes, and you will hear that women are more likely to attend church, to take their faith very seriously, and to put into practice their concern for others, especially other women and children. Scholars of religion, like Janet Liebman Jacobs (2002), Nancy Ammerman (2006), and Meredith McGuire (2008), to name but a few, refer to the concept of lived religion – the religious or spiritual practices that characterize daily life.[3] Lived religion highlights what women do in their homes, in their kitchens, in their workplaces, and in their social lives that brings faith and religious traditions to the fore. Themes of freedom, justice, choice, and agency find their way into the everyday experiences of women as they live in family and work together in the broader culture. As we shall see, abuse limits women's freedom, the justice they seek, and the choices open to them, yet even in these limiting circumstances, agency still operates. To characterize women connected with churches across Canada and beyond as strong spirits is simply to give voice to what is obvious to both religious and secular commentators.

Abuse of women's bodies happens inside and beyond communities of faith.[4] Women who are beautiful, women who are rich, women who are educated, women who are poor, and women who are strong of spirit can be – and are – victimized by the men they have promised to love until death draws them apart. This is especially hard for many people to believe and to accept as fact. Both men and women find the statistics overwhelming.[5] Those who have grown up with the reality of abuse sometimes have little patience with the lack of understanding that is so pervasive concerning domestic violence. Resistance to the data on abuse takes a variety of forms. Sometimes, it is a "not in my backyard" reaction, where those who are educated or of substantial financial means find it difficult to accept that others who share these characteristics with them can participate in such heinous activities. Nowhere is this notion stronger than among the highly religious.

When deeply committed Christian women are abused, they are highly vulnerable. There are several reasons for this. Religious women as a group also confront some unique needs as they journey toward healing and wholeness. I shall expand on both of these points by offering a case illustration from my fieldwork.

Mildred and Russell Jennings[6] might have looked like a happy couple at church, but at home things were very volatile. Russell's desire for power and status led to purchases they could not afford, and the mounting debt set the tone for angst at home. To outsiders, it appeared that the couple had everything – successful adult children, flashy cars, and a lovely home – but their economic woes were hidden just like the violence. Russell gave very little thought to Mildred or her needs. Mildred was caught between attempting to satisfy the demands of her husband and the very pressing needs of her elderly mother, who lived with them. Shy and retiring, Mildred's response to Russell was to try very hard to please him. He wanted to control her life as much as possible, including where she went and with whom. When she resisted his control, he would adopt one of two strategies: refuse to speak at all or yell and call her names. On one occasion, he attempted to kill her.

As a very spiritual woman, Mildred felt it was her religious duty to forgive Russell "seventy times seven," following what she believed the scriptures taught.[7] She suffered from low self-esteem, which had been compounded, no doubt, by watching her father lash out against her mother within her childhood home – a pattern that she had observed between her maternal grandparents as well.

Mildred sought the help of her pastor when Russell forced both women from the home – giving them two hours' notice to leave and never return. Within hours of her call for help, the pastor found temporary shelter for these two older women with another church family who owned a large farmhouse in the countryside.

As the days progressed, Mildred had so many unanswered questions. What was God expecting of her now? Would she ever be forgiven for leaving Russell? Should she go back to him now? The pastor helped Mildred to recognize her misguided religious convictions regarding forgiveness and marriage. He walked alongside her, even as he challenged the faulty beliefs that caused her to feel guilty and experience remorse. In time, she was able to see that God did not require her to ignore the abusive treatment she had received but rather to hold her husband accountable for his actions and his words. The pastor acted as a mediator between Mildred's spiritual angst and her very practical problems. He helped legal counsel to understand why Mildred was so forgiving of her husband, and he offered a spiritual supplement to the advice and support that she was receiving from community-based workers. By helping her to negotiate her faith and ongoing need for safety and housing, he offered a bridge between her strong spirit and her abused body. In spiritual terms, he became the answer to her prayer.

A repeated theme arising in my fieldwork over the years has been the primacy of spiritual issues on the road to healing and wholeness for those religious women whose lives have been impacted by domestic violence. Like Mildred, they felt like a shattered window when violence robbed them of peace and safety at home. Like Mildred, they had placed the intact family in high regard, believing that they had made a promise to God that they would never turn their back on the marriage. Like Mildred, they felt that they needed to keep on forgiving, to keep on suffering, to keep on trying to salvage the marriage, and to keep on hoping – and believing – that the violence would end and that their partner would change his abusive ways.

Through my research, I have learned that most religious women who are abused do not believe that the term "battered wife" applies to them. Julie Owens, a nationally recognized domestic violence advocate, and herself a battered wife, tells the story of how, after her husband was sent to prison for attempting to murder her (and her father), she heard on the radio of a program in Hawaii for battered wives and called to see whether she might attend. She said to the domestic violence advocate on the phone, "I am not a battered wife, but my husband tried to kill me."[8]

In contrast to the nonreligious, not only do very religious women conceptualize their own abuse differently, but they also seek out different sources of assistance in its aftermath. Often they are skeptical of secular sources of help, fearing that they have let down the faith community by declaring the violence to "nonbelievers." Also, they are especially prone to feel that if they had been truly spiritual, the violence would not have happened. Often they experience both the fear and reality of rejection by some members of their congregational community when failure of the marriage becomes known. As a result, many religious women place a lot of confidence in any assistance that can be offered to their abusive partners: "If only he would seek help."

In part, the enthusiasm among religious survivors of domestic violence for various kinds of batterer intervention directed toward abusive husbands prompted me to begin research to see whether there was any evidence of changed behaviour among those who had been participants in a faith-based, state-certified program for abusive men. To introduce some of the features of this work, I begin with the story of one couple seeking help from a faith-based agency I studied with colleague Barbara Fisher-Townsend.[9]

Pablo and Nala began to look for help when the Department of Human Services (DHS) in the northwestern US state where they resided took their little girl from their home and placed her in foster care. In the whirlwind of emotion that followed, Nala heard about the local faith-based program for families experiencing domestic violence from her DHS worker. She acted immediately on the referral suggestion and contacted the program. According to Pablo, "We decided that we don't want this to, I guess, continue ... DV [domestic violence] in our relationship because I am not a woman beater and she is not a man beater and we had a very unfortunate incident happen in our house and we wanted to correct that."[10]

The "incident" of domestic violence, as Pablo was prone to call it, was witnessed by their eighteen-month-old daughter, and when the police were called, the DHS became involved because there was physical evidence that the child might have been mistreated. Pablo and Nala were suspected of child abuse, and their daughter was removed from their care.

Adamant that they had not harmed their child, but forthright about the domestic violence in their relationship as a couple, Pablo and Nala were determined to regain custody of their daughter. They were young, vulnerable, working-class Latinos residing in a region of the United States that was not very ethnically diverse. They were extremely worried about what would happen to them and to their little girl. "So me and my wife decided we are going to try to satisfy DHS, enrol ourselves, get help for what happened way back then, and just continue this course of bettering ourselves ... So I am here mainly to try to get my daughter back. We know nobody hurt our child, but they don't, so they want us to attend these [parenting] classes." Simultaneous to their involvement with the intervention programs and personal counselling at the faith-based agency, Nala sought help from her pastor for all their troubles. Pablo accompanied her. They went for pastoral counselling and received training related to family life.

Pablo's background was challenging: his father was an alcoholic who earned extra cash playing pool. "Actually he made most of his money going to the bars because he was a pool shark and he would come home with money, you know, but at the same time he would be drunk, so we would have to see Mom and Dad argue all the time ... loud enough for four kids to get scared." In elementary school, in the southern United States, Pablo learned early that "if you aren't one of the bullies, then you are one of the ones getting bullied." He had a "history of constant fighting." He even pursued fighting as a sport: "I love boxing on punching bags and stuff like that, just for the exercise of it." As a teen, he possessed an athletic body, played on multiple sport teams, and harboured the attitude of a fighter.

From his early days of involvement with the faith-based batterer intervention program, Pablo appeared very enthusiastic about gaining insight into his own behaviour, his past, and his intimate relationship with Nala. However, he remained focused on his primary goal: the return of their daughter to live with them together as a family. He spoke of change and of God: "I don't think anybody can really change without Him. That's my belief ... You know, do whatever works for you, but definitely look at yourself for a minute 'cause if you don't, then you will never really know what you are." Crisis in his life heightened Pablo's interest in his spiritual side. Pablo said, "I have always believed in God, but I never believed in it wholeheartedly, and now I believe a little bit more stronger. I have never been a crier and when this happened with my daughter, I prayed to God and I just busted out in tears, so I definitely feel there is somebody listening to me."

Like many abusive men whom Fisher-Townsend and I have studied, Pablo drinks to excess: "You know, alcohol is a downer, it just ruins everybody's life pretty much, so I am not invisible to it and it's got its hands on me and obviously it came back to bite me in the rear end ... I am not untouchable." Raised Catholic by a father who practised his faith and a mother who was rather indifferent to hers, Pablo found comfort and support from his Christian background even though he never embraced it wholeheartedly. "I don't like to play two-faced, but I like the words, I like the words from the Bible, and that is what he [their pastor] preaches to me, so I love to hear it ... And the book we study on the secret to family happiness and everything that's in there, the Bible backs up, so I believe it. If it was coming from somebody's mouth that had a hunch, I would be like ummm, you know, it doesn't sit well in my stomach."

Pablo was very enthusiastic about how the facilitator integrated spiritual content into the batterer intervention groups. In his words, she did a "really good job with trying not to offend people that don't believe in God. She will quote a scripture from the Bible every now and then, but she won't push God onto anybody ... She has it memorized and that is about it. I think it's just enough so that it won't scare somebody away that doesn't believe or make them mad or upset ... If you can have backup, it might as well be God."

From Pablo's point of view, the intervention helped him to remain "violent-free" through this very stressful period of their daughter in foster care. He joked, "I am telling you, if my brothers, or someone, has a problem, I could probably repair it for them right there on the phone ... I have learned a lot and with the stress that me and my wife are going through right now, I think without the tools that I have, I would have crumbled a long time ago ... I got plenty of tools on me now."

Despite the tools that he had been acquiring, Pablo admitted that he could get angry pretty easily; he had "one of those short fuses." But "with all the help that I am getting and all the people in my life, all of a sudden, I think I am able to address things easier and keep it calm instead of boiling. I am warm." But whether warm was cool enough, only time would reveal.

With an army of workers offering them support, Nala and Pablo were staying the course. He was in a drug rehabilitation program and a batterer intervention group, they attended a parenting class together, both were engaged in individual psychotherapy, Nala met with the DHS worker on a regular basis, and they both met weekly with their pastor. The supervised visitation took place at church; the elder of the congregation brought their daughter from the foster family to visit with them at church. After the service, the elder returned the little girl to the foster home. Pablo and Nala saw their daughter on two other occasions per week, bringing their total hours of weekly visitation to four. The elder came to their home each week and met with the facilitator of the parenting program once a month and, less often, with the social worker at the DHS. He was certainly committed to a community response to Pablo and Nala's problems and willing to see himself as part of the solution to the angst they were facing.

In six months' time, we interviewed Pablo again. We learned that the child had been returned to Nala on the condition that Nala and Pablo live apart. Although they complied with the DHS order, it was causing them financial strain. Pablo was allowed to see their daughter in supervised contexts. He was not allowed to visit with her at Nala's place of residence.

As a result of the cost of keeping two separate living spaces, Pablo had decided to move in with his parents. Probably this was causing some strain with his parents, an older couple who had already endured some of the difficulties of Pablo's wayward past.

He interjected here about his prison time – something that he had denied on our first visit (although we knew from the file analysis that he had been in trouble with the law before). In prison – a result of four convictions for driving while impaired – he had learned some new skills, had earned his general education diploma, and had become certified as a plumber and a drywaller.

We learned that a year out of penitentiary, Pablo had met Nala. After six months in the batterer intervention program, Pablo was still committed to the program and its goals. He was attending classes, working at the same job, and hoping that soon he would be reunited with his family. Using the mantra from Alcoholics Anonymous of "one day at a time," Pablo noted that if he stayed the course and fulfilled all the obligations, this reunion would happen, he just needed to be patient: "One day at a time is that tool belt that I am adding together." Like many men we have interviewed, reunification with his daughter was a strong incentive to stay the course and do the work that was necessary for changed thinking and changed behaviour. But this course was extremely challenging for him to maintain.

When we returned one year later to interview Pablo again, he was not available to see us. He had gone back to drinking, and Nala had taken their child and gone back to Texas. The couple was seeking a divorce. The family would not be reunited. His drinking and his violence had not been curtailed. Only his resolve to change had been altered.

Social, Political, and Theological Reflections

Fear is a primary aspect of domestic violence. First and foremost, there is the victim's fear. In her book *Battered Wives,* Del Martin (1981) argues that fear is the primary reason why women do not leave husbands who abuse them. A battered wife fears for her safety and the safety of her children. She fears reprisal if she tells someone of the horror she is living. She fears the future, and the paralyzing terror she experiences can impact her waking hours as well as her sleep. In fact, fear in many ways is responsible for keeping an abused woman from making choices that would enhance her personal safety.[11] Covering up the story of abuse – for fear of being found out – also takes a lot of energy, which could otherwise be directed to making plans for leaving the relationship and ensuring safety for all.

However, fear is also a component of why pastors and other religious leaders do not speak out against domestic violence in a way that they could – or might be encouraged to do. My research among clergy has revealed that many are reluctant to preach against violence at home for *fear* of what will happen the next week as victims, survivors, perpetrators, and family members contact them. Sometimes it is a matter of being very poorly equipped, educationally speaking, to respond to the cries for help. Sometimes it is a matter of not knowing how or when to refer those parishioners who need help beyond the expertise of the pastor. Sometimes it is a fear of referrals themselves, based on the idea that the advice of a domestic violence advocate, or a lawyer, or a therapist will be damaging to a woman's faith. As psychologist Victoria Fahlberg (Nason-Clark et al. 2010) has argued, religious leaders who fear that a referral will jeopardize a woman's spiritual journey have very little trust in the woman herself or her judgment. She argues that whether they will lose their faith in the institutional church depends more on how they are treated by the congregation and its leadership than on what they hear at a secular agency about their faith. Sometimes, too, a victim of domestic violence does not want to seek assistance outside of her faith community for fear of having her faith ridiculed. Sometimes, however, a religious victim does not want to seek help within her faith community for fear of rejection or compromised confidentiality, among other factors.[12]

Reluctance on the part of clergy to refer survivors or perpetrators for help is an interesting phenomenon. Research has revealed that referrals are least likely to occur where they are needed most: among those clergy with very little knowledge of – and experience in responding to – domestic violence (Whipple 1987; Horton and Williamson 1988; Weaver 1993; Kroeger and Nason-Clark 2010). This reluctance put lives at risk.

In an effort to understand some of the issues surrounding referrals more clearly, I organized an invited panel of clergy and community personnel to discuss the nature and dynamics of the referral process at a conference in 2008 in Washington, DC, and later published some of the highlights (Nason-Clark et al. 2010; see also Nason-Clark 1997).[13] To contextualize the issues, I offered a few pieces of empirical evidence related to referrals from ongoing research. First, in one study of 343 evangelical clergy, I learned that 15 percent had never made a referral suggestion for professional help on any issue over the years of their ministry. Of those who had referred, 39 percent had done so in fewer than one in ten cases that involved relationship or marriage matters (including abuse). At the other end of the spectrum, 14 percent of pastors had referred in at least half of the cases that had come to them for relationship counselling. Fewer than one in ten clergy, or 8 percent, reported that they were well equipped to respond to the needs of those who sought their help in the aftermath of domestic violence.

In another study involving interviews with 100 conservative Protestant pastors, my colleagues and I (Nason-Clark 1997; Kroeger and Nason-Clark 2010) learned that the average minister spends 16 percent of his or her time counselling parishioners (two afternoons a week) and that it is considered by men and women in ministry to be the most stressful part of their work. The most frequently cited reason among clergy for suggesting a referral resource is their own feeling of personal inadequacy to respond to the individual seeking help. Interestingly, most clergy report that they are satisfied with the counsel received by parishioners who follow through on clerical advice to seek the help of a secular counsellor.

Over the years of research, I have learned that there are a number of factors that shape pastoral counselling strategies and a pastor's willingness or reluctance to make referrals to professionals in the community or to community-based agencies. One that may come as a surprise is the role of personal experience with help-seeking behaviour on the part of clergy counsellors or a member of their immediate family. Another relates to whether counselling is viewed as effective by those clergy who are most experienced at offering it. Interestingly, it is clerical attitudes about counselling, rather than the level of training to offer it, that seem to distinguish pastors from one another. Experienced counsellors are less pessimistic about the difficulties associated with referring a parishioner to a secular counsellor for help, and they are far more knowledgeable about what resources are actually available in their local area. These religious leaders make their referral suggestions based on their knowledge of the person and on their counselling or professional skills rather than on the faith perspective of the referral resource. Moreover, pastors with more extensive referral networks are able to outline the specific role of the pastoral counsellor in a co-ordinated community response, likely in part because they have personally been challenged by their own networking opportunities to think through their own particularity. These clergy also talk far more explicitly about the spiritual emphasis of their own counselling. Because of this emphasis, they are able to contribute to a co-ordinated community response in ways that many other religious leaders might not.

From the perspective of a religious leader, one of the most significant factors in making referrals to community agencies and secular professionals is the lack of relationships with people in these agencies.[14] If you do not know the people at the local women's shelter or know the local advocates for victims of domestic violence and if you have few contacts with secular agencies in the community, it is very difficult to make a referral suggestion or to help a parishioner make this contact. For referrals, however, the problem is not only that clergy may not trust secular agencies but also that the workers at these agencies may not trust religious leaders.

From the perspective of an agency director, churches don't take abuse seriously enough because it is often kept hidden by the victims and offenders.[15] As a result, church leaders and their congregations are often unaware of how pervasive, dangerous, and harmful domestic violence is within their congregations and the broader society. Lacking training, clergy – particularly of a theologically right-leaning persuasion – often resort to traditional theological positions related to family relationships, such as male entitlement, female submission, and prohibitions on divorce.

Moreover, since outrage over domestic violence came out of the secular feminist movement, and since feminism has been so demonized by some in religious circles (and vice versa), anything coming from the feminist movement is automatically suspect. That some domestic violence advocates may see religious traditions and their sacred writings as irrelevant, or even harmful, poses a challenge for any co-operative working arrangement between the so-called secular and the sacred. Of course, religious institutions too often want to solve everything within their own walls, no matter what the problem. Turning or referring to an outside secular agency is viewed by some pastors as "failing" their congregants. This fear of failure can motivate an untrained pastor to refuse to include others in the community as part of a collaborative team to help a church family in the aftermath of domestic violence.

Fear concerning domestic violence also extends to the seminary. In one study involving four seminaries and over 400 seminary students, Steve McMullin and I learned that of the 66 graduating students among our participants,[16] fewer than one in ten, or 7.6 percent, felt that they were well prepared to respond to situations of domestic violence in their ministry. This figure contrasts with 4.9 percent of the 364 students (not yet in their graduating year) who reported that they felt well prepared to respond. As can be seen, there was only a slight improvement in students' self-assessment of their preparedness to respond to cases of abuse as they approached graduation from the seminary. It is noteworthy that nearly half of the graduating students still believed that they were either poorly prepared or not prepared at all.

Despite the considerable geographic, theological, and doctrinal differences among the seminaries, the students in all four educational institutions estimated the extent of domestic violence in families within congregations (25.0%) to be lower than in families in the wider society (34.1%). The good news of these data is that students did in fact realize that abuse was widespread – but they were unequivocal that it occurred with less frequency in families of faith. When you combine this data with their own self-assessment of a lack of preparation for ministry in this area, it becomes clear why one of the important themes that emerged from the student focus groups was fear about addressing and responding to domestic violence in the future. As a group, they lacked knowledge about community-based resources (e.g., 55.5 percent did not know how to contact a transition house). Female students as a group felt better prepared than male students, and married students felt better prepared than single students, but the most significant factor in raising students' self-assessment on preparation was whether they had ever visited a shelter for battered women.

In focus group discussions, sometimes the fear expressed by many students about responding to issues of abuse in their future ministries was personal ("It just scares me"), and sometimes it was a fear that if they raised the issue in a sermon, victims would come for help, and "you're not ready for it." Others were fearful that the ministry of the church could be destroyed by disclosures, and still others were fearful of the extent or pervasiveness of abuse among those in their churches: "[Is it] ... okay if a spouse is verbally abusive? ... Do we let them serve on the committee? Where do we draw the line?" The students had lots of questions that needed to be addressed in the seminary classroom by an instructor familiar both with church traditions and with the subject of abuse.

What this seminary study has revealed is that fear is intertwined with how seminary students understand domestic violence. They are fearful about addressing it in a congregational context and fearful about responding to those who seek their help after it occurs. Sometimes this fear is based on their own narrative, sometimes it is caused by a gap between the training they believe they need and the seminary's ability to provide it, and sometimes it is linked to a concern that they may thwart the healing journey of a survivor by doing or saying the wrong thing. With limited experience or knowledge related to the topic of abuse, many seminary students have reason to be fearful. Yet these data reveal that having knowledge of resources and a familiarity with referral sources reduces the fear that seminarians report.

Since fear seems to permeate so many aspects of domestic violence work, it seems important to consider how putting in place safety measures and support structures might realistically reduce this fear. The stories of Mildred and Nala, told above, give us some clues. The strong social support structure that can be offered by congregational life is key. In Mildred's case, it was a religious leader who heard her cries for help and offered simultaneously practical support and spiritual guidance. He found Mildred and her mother temporary lodging in a safe place, and then he began to address her spiritual questions and religious angst. Acting as a bridge between her faith and the referral options in the community (specifically her lawyer), the pastor explained religious behaviour to a secular professional even as he directly challenged Mildred's erroneous religious ideation in counselling with her.

Here, themes of freedom, justice, choice, and agency emerge from what might be considered the fog of erroneous religious rhetoric. Several chapters in this volume discuss these themes. Catherine Holtmann and Heather Shipley, in particular, highlight the chasm between rhetoric and reality, as do Pamela Dickey Young, Andrew Kam-Tuck Yip, and Tracy Trothen. Studying the lives of real people – in all of their complexities – as they personally mediate the somewhat porous boundaries between the sacred and the secular reveals that explanations that rely on the secularization thesis or, for that matter, on any unitary explanation simply do not account in any meaningful way for how religion intersects in women's and men's daily lives. In Mildred's case, it was a religious leader who mediated the challenging pathway – her case illustrates one strategy that an abused religious woman, who was strong in spirit, employed in an attempt to work out her own personal journey (replete with choices, agency, and challenges) as an abused body with a strong spiritual identity.

In the case of Pablo and Nala, a religious elder negotiated the practical challenges of the transfer of their child from foster care to supervised visitation, which occurred in the church building. At the same time, their religious leader helped them to see there was hope that their daughter could be returned if they did the work that was required, such as Pablo joining the batterer intervention group and entering the drug rehabilitation program, as well as Nala and Pablo together going to parenting classes. Using the language of their faith tradition, the leader supported Nala's desire to ensure that Pablo received the help he needed, even as she recognized that counselling would assist her to gain strength and to bring her daughter home. When it became clear to Nala that despite the intervention of a faith-based agency and her pastor, Pablo was unwilling – or unable – to change, she took action by leaving the state where Pablo's probabation mandated that he remain and by taking the child with her.

Here, too, we see the co-mingling of religious and secular frameworks to offer a way forward that is sensitive both to the language of the faith community of which the woman is a part and to a broader cultural narrative of safety and respite for women and their dependent children in the aftermath of domestic violence. When it became clear to the religious leader that Nala and Pablo could not be reunited – that her safety would be compromised and the child put at risk – notions of family togetherness, so important to the faith tradition, were held to be subservient to notions of the sanctity and centrality of the preservation of human life. Here, there was both a religious and secular imperative to keep Nala and her child safe. For this purpose, the celebration of family life – a religious motif – was interpreted to mean the safety of mother and child.

Through interviews with criminal justice workers, as well as therapeutic staff and domestic violence advocates, I have learned how different their paradigms and understandings concerning matters of marriage and the family can be from those of clergy and other religious leaders. Yet, when there is respect and a mutual desire to reduce domestic violence and its impact, collaboration between secular and religious agents becomes a way to bridge the chasm between a woman's strong spirit and her abused body. Using spiritual language to talk about a theology of suffering, about the empowerment of a survivor through her relation with a personal God, about an ethic of compassion in congregational life, and about the call to social justice helps a religious woman to negotiate her identity as a woman of faith, as a *strong spirit,* and as a body that has been broken and abused. In this way, her religious identity offers strength amid the crisis, and the religious resources of her congregational community and faith tradition help to augment her journey toward healing and wholeness.

Concluding Comments

The impact of domestic violence on families of faith has social, political, and theological undertones. Several chapters in this volume highlight the constraints of framing religious identity as prescribing a *lived experience* of rigid, inflexible, unchanging gender or sexual narratives, orientations, or dynamics that impact the way one thinks and the way one acts. Violence in families of faith offers an example of how truly nuanced and interwoven are the dynamics of faith, gender, and sexuality when violence strikes at home. Certainly, there are patterns to be observed. Certainly, there are elements of the religious and elements of the secular. However, in individual cases, the web of connections between sex, gender, culture, violence, and faith needs to be understood both from the perspective of the person who has been violated and in terms of the larger network of people who assist on the journey toward justice, accountability, healing, and wholeness.

Navigating the relatively uncharted waters of *both* the religious and the secular implications of an abused body and a strong spirit is critical for those who seek to understand, as well as for those who support, families impacted by domestic violence. The cases discussed in this chapter illustrate *the reality of fear* but also the power and complexity of human agency, *the reality of control* but also the power of those who are prepared and trained to assist, and the *centrality of faith* – through its leaders and the traditions they represent – to mediate and negotiate strategies that take into account some of the social, political, and theological issues facing those impacted when abuse occurs in the domestic realm. In so doing, these cases blur the boundaries between the secular and the religious by showing that those who have been victimized seek to reclaim their lives with the help of both secular and religious agents who are willing to walk alongside them on the road to peace and safety.

Notes

I gratefully acknowledge the agencies that have funded my research program over the past twenty years, including the Louisville Institute for the Study of Protestantism and American Culture, the Social Sciences and Humanities Research Council of Canada, the Lawson Foundation, and most recently, the Lilly Endowment, which provided a five-year grant to enable the development of the Religion and Violence e-Learning (RAVE) Project for religious leaders. This project's resources can be accessed at http://www.theraveproject.org.

1 I am especially indebted to the work of Catherine Clark Kroeger (Kroeger and Beck 1996, 1998) and Marie Fortune (Fortune 1987, 1991) for highlighting the many and varied ways that religious women are overcomers (see also Clarke 1986; Giesbrecht and Sevcik 2000; Stirling et al. 2004; Clark Kroeger, Nason-Clark, and Fisher-Townsend 2008; and Popesciu et al. 2009).

2 In one project involving focus groups with a large number of conservative Protestant women (N = 247), these issues were highlighted. They were then confirmed in later research that included interviews with individual women or pastors (N = 194) (see Nason-Clark 1997, 2004, 2009).

3 Jacobs (2002) and McGuire (2008) note that women often use food preparation and the enjoyment of food with their families as part of their religious service or as a religious act.

4 For a fuller review of this issue, consult Kroeger and Nason-Clark (2010); for incidence rates, see Statistics Canada (2008) and DeKeseredy and MacLeod (1998); for an earlier review of abuse and religion, see Horton and Williamson (1988); and for an overview of some of the theological issues, consult Fiorenza and Copeland (1994) and Brown and Bohn (1989).

5 According to data collected by Statistics Canada (2005), 653,000 Canadian women had reported being a victim of spousal violence in the previous five years. A staggering 26 percent of these Canadian women had been assaulted more than ten times. The violence experienced in Canada by women at the hands of their intimate partners tends to be more severe – and repeated more often – than the abuse experienced by men. Violence within intimate relationships is highest among the young, with women between the ages of fifteen and twenty-four reporting the highest one-year rates of such abuse.

6 These names are fictitious, and some of the details of Mildred's story have been altered slightly to protect her identity. Portions of her story have been told in Nason-Clark and Kroeger (2004) and in Kroeger and Nason-Clark (2010).
7 "Seventy times seven" refers to the words of Jesus to the disciples when they asked how often someone should forgive another (Matthew 18:22). It has been taken to mean: more times than the number of transgressions.
8 Based on a presentation by Julie Owens at an international PASCH [Peace and Safety in the Christian Home] Conference, Newport Beach, California, 25 February 2006 (see Owens 2008).
9 My account of this couple's story is adapted from work in progress on *Men Who Batter,* a book co-authored with Barbara Fisher-Townsend for Oxford University Press; for a fuller explanation of our ongoing research on abusive men, see Fisher-Townsend et al. (2008). Portions of this story also appear in Nason-Clark et al. (2013).
10 These verbatim quotations are from interviews I conducted between 2005 and 2009.
11 Both Janet Jakobsen and Tracy Trothen in this volume discuss systemic factors that impinge on one's agency.
12 See the results of research conducted in Calgary by Sevcik et al. (2011).
13 The following few paragraphs summarize portions of the panel presentation and the publication based on it.
14 Here, I summarize Steve McMullin's contribution in Nason-Clark et al. (2010).
15 Here, I summarize Victoria Fahlberg's contribution in Nason-Clark et al. (2010).
16 The following three paragraphs summarize some of the findings to appear in McMullin and Nason-Clark (2011).

References

Ammerman, N.T. 2006. *Everyday Religion: Observing Modern Religious Lives.* New York: Oxford University Press.

Brown, J., and C. Bohn. 1989. *Christianity, Patriarchy and Abuse: A Feminist Critique.* Cleveland: Pilgrim.

Clarke, R.L. 1986. *Pastoral Care of Battered Women.* Philadelphia: Westminster.

DeKeseredy, W., and L. MacLeod. 1998. *Woman Abuse: A Sociological Story.* Toronto: Harcourt Brace.

Fiorenza, E.S., and M.S. Copeland, eds. 1994. *Violence against Women.* London: SCM Press.

Fisher-Townsend, B., N. Nason-Clark, L. Ruff, and N. Murphy. 2008. I Am Not Violent: Men's Experience in Group. In *Beyond Abuse in the Christian Home: Raising Voices for Change,* ed. C. Clark Kroeger, N. Nason-Clark, and B. Fisher-Townsend, 78-99. Eugene, OR: Wipf and Stock.

Fortune, M. 1987. *Keeping the Faith: Questions and Answers for the Abused Woman.* San Francisco: Harper.

–. 1991. *Violence in the Family: A Workshop Curriculum for Clergy and Other Helpers.* Cleveland: Pilgrim.

Giesbrecht, N., and I. Sevcik. 2000. The Process of Recovery and Rebuilding among Abused Women in Conservative Evangelical Subculture. *Journal of Family Violence* 15 (3): 229-48.

Horton, A., and J. Williamson. 1988. *Abuse and Religion: When Praying Isn't Enough.* New York: D.C. Heath.

Jacobs, J.L. 2002. *Hidden Heritage: The Legacy of the Crypto-Jews.* Berkeley: University of California Press.

Kroeger, C. Clark, and J. Beck, eds. 1996. *Woman, Abuse and the Bible: How Scripture Can Be Used to Hurt or to Heal.* Grand Rapids, MI: Baker.

–, eds. 1998. *Healing the Hurting: Giving Hope and Help to Abused Women.* Grand Rapids, MI: Baker.

Kroeger, C. Clark, and N. Nason-Clark. 2010. *No Place for Abuse: Biblical and Practical Resources to Counteract Domestic Violence.* 2nd ed. Downers Grove, IL: InterVarsity.

Kroeger, C. Clark, N. Nason-Clark, and B. Fisher-Townsend, eds. 2008. *Beyond Abuse in the Christian Home: Raising Voices for Change.* Eugene, OR: Wipf and Stock.

Martin, Del. 1981. *Battered Wives.* San Francisco: New Glide.

McGuire, M.B. 2008. *Lived Religion: Faith and Practice in Everyday Life.* New York: Oxford University Press.

McMullin, S., and N. Nason-Clark. 2011. Equipping Seminary Students to Respond to Abuse: A Look at the Research. In *Responding to Abuse in Christian Homes: A Challenge to Churches and Their Leaders,* ed. N. Nason-Clark, C. Clark Kroeger, and B. Fisher-Townsend, 231-46. Eugene, OR: Wipf and Stock.

Nason-Clark, N. 1997. *The Battered Wife: How Christians Confront Family Violence.* Louisville, KY: Westminster John Knox Press.

–. 2000. Making the Sacred Safe: Woman Abuse and Communities of Faith. *Sociology of Religion* 61 (4): 349-68.

–. 2004. When Terror Strikes at Home: The Interface between Religion and Domestic Violence. *Journal for the Scientific Study of Religion* 42 (3): 303-10.

–. 2009. Christianity and the Experience of Domestic Violence: What Does Faith Have to Do with It? *Christianity and Social Work* 36 (4): 379-93.

–. 2013. Talking about Domestic Violence and Communities of Faith in the Public Sphere: Celebrations and Challenges. In *Religion in the Public Sphere: Interdisciplinary Perspectives across the Canadian Provinces,* ed. S. Lefevre and L. Beaman, 149-70. Toronto: University of Toronto Press.

Nason-Clark, N., B. Fisher-Townsend, S. McMullin, and C. Holtmann. 2013. Life Stories of Men Who Act Abusively: Elements of the Coordinated Community Response. In *Strengthening Families and Ending Abuse: Churches and Their Leaders Look to the Future,* ed. N. Nason-Clark, B. Fisher-Townsend, and V. Fahlberg, 40-64. Eugene, OR: Wipf and Stock.

Nason-Clark, N., and C. Clark Kroeger. 2004. *Refuge from Abuse: Hope and Healing for Abused Christian Women*. Downers Grove, IL: InterVarsity.

Nason-Clark, N., S. McMullin, V. Fahlberg, and D. Schaefer. 2010. Referrals between Clergy and Community-Based Resources: Challenges and Opportunities. *Journal of Family and Community Ministries* 23 (4): 10-20.

Owens, J. 2008. A Survivor Looks Back: What I Wish Pastors Had Known When I Was Looking for Help. In *Beyond Abuse in the Christian Home: Raising Voices for Change*, ed. C. Clark Kroeger, N. Nason-Clark, and B. Fisher-Townsend, 2-23. Eugene, OR: Wipf and Stock.

Popesciu, M., R. Drumm, S. Mayer, L. Cooper, T. Foster, M. Seifert, H. Gadd, and S. Dewan. 2009. "Because of my beliefs that I had acquired from the church ...": Religious Belief-Based Barriers for Adventist Women in Domestic Violence Relationships. *Christianity and Social Work* 36 (4): 394-414.

Sevcik, I., N. Nason-Clark, M. Rothery, and R. Pynn. 2011. Finding Their Voices and Speaking Out: Research amongst Women of Faith in Western Canada. In *Responding to Abuse in Christian Homes: A Challenge to Churches and Their Leaders*, ed. N. Nason-Clark, C. Clark Kroeger, and B. Fisher-Townsend, 169-89. Eugene, OR: Wipf and Stock.

Statistics Canada. 2005. *Family Violence in Canada: A Statistical Profile*. Ottawa: Canadian Centre for Justice Statistics.

–. 2008. *Family Violence in Canada: A Statistical Profile*. Ottawa: Canadian Centre for Justice Statistics.

Stirling, M.L., C.A. Cameron, N. Nason-Clark, and B. Miedema. 2004. *Understanding Abuse: Partnering for Change*. Toronto: University of Toronto Press.

Weaver, A.J. 1993. Psychological Trauma: What Clergy Need to Know. *Pastoral Psychology* 41 (6): 385-408.

Whipple, V. 1987. Counseling Battered Women from Fundamentalist Churches. *Journal for Marital and Family Therapy* 13 (3): 251-58.

Conclusion

Pamela Dickey Young

The authors in this volume were brought together by an interest in the academic study of religion and sexuality and by a desire to challenge the idea that the link between religion and sexuality is a relatively simple one, where religion's power is used to uphold certain views of sexuality that the religious deem appropriate. Certainly, this reading is true in some instances, especially where official religious institutions get involved in public policy debates (e.g., Dickey Young, Lee, Shipley, and Holtmann, this volume). But the reality is so much more complex than this simple reading. As individuals appropriate and construct their own religiosities and sexualities, the breadth of the relationships between varied forms of religion and varied sexualities becomes astonishing (e.g., Yip, Holtmann, Boisvert, Trothen, and Nason-Clark, this volume). Neither religion nor sexuality is singular and monolithic. Groups and individuals have mobilized religion both to mandate "approved sexualities" and to validate a wider variety of sexualities. Interestingly enough, as Jakobsen points out in Chapter 1, the notion of approved sexualities, even when not restricted to straight sexualities, can still be problematic because people are then categorized according to whether they fit some specific norm, meaning that there are always others who are continually placed outside this norm.

Common themes arose in the process of constructing this volume. The authors whose work appears here share an inclination that the rhetoric and the actions of tolerance and accommodation are not sufficiently robust approaches either to religious diversity or to sexual diversity. To continue to use this rhetoric and these actions is to assume both a norm for sexuality and religion and an "other" who must be tolerated or accommodated. In the case of the geographic locales investigated in this volume, the religious norm is Christianity and the sexual norm is heterosexual marriage. Reimagining what could exist beyond tolerance and accommodation is a thematic strand in this volume, especially as this reimagining extends to lived religions of whatever sort that might well differ from the norms of organized religious groups. Even though the reimaginings do not all take the same form, the desire to move beyond the dominant model for dealing with diversity is common across the chapters.

Another common theme in this volume is a puzzlement over why sex has been the site of so much angst – religious angst and cultural angst – particularly, for this collection, within North America and the United Kingdom. Education systems, social policy makers, religious groups, and sports regulators all seem to have bought into the notion that sexuality is a public/social problem that needs to be fretted over and "solved." Although this has not always been the case (see Jakobsen, Chapter 1, this volume), sexuality causes moral panic in North American and British society in ways that, for example, economics does not. The authors of this volume highlight a variety of ways that religion and sex are linked together in the public imagination, most of which involve the "public" seeing religion as one appropriate means of regulating sexuality. But as many of the chapters imply, this construction assumes a dominant and monolithic "public." As soon as one begins to look at individual religiosity (e.g., Yip, Holtmann, Boisvert, Trothen, and Nason-Clark, this volume), one sees that religion and sexuality are related in complex ways. If one thinks of sexuality only as the "problem" and of religion only as the "solution," this discounts the way that many religious people actually live their lives, and it ignores the lives of countless sexual minority persons (religious and otherwise) who resist having their lives construed as problematic. The authors in this book ask what is to be counted as public space and who, in the public, gets to determine how this space will be understood and regulated.

All of the book's authors – although not all of their research interlocutors (e.g., Yip, Holtmann, and Nason-Clark) – understand religion and sexuality as social constructions. Religion and sexuality are "queer" in that they are unstable and fluid. The construction of a religious or sexual identity (or of the two intersecting identities together) is a multifaceted interaction between religious and other social forces and the agency of any given individual. This identity is not always stable over time. It can change in response to a variety of forces. There are pervasive hegemonic forces that seek to control both sexual and religious identities. In North America and the United Kingdom, certain forms of Christianity provide the religious hegemonic forces, and the hegemonic sexual force is toward heteronormatvity. In Canada, Christian hegemony is a combination of Protestant and Roman Catholic hegemonies (see Beaman 2003), in the United States it is characterized by Calvinism (see Jakobsen, Chapter 1, this volume), and in the United Kingdom it is the purview of the Church of England. Nonetheless, people regularly construct their sexual and religious identities in ways that differ from those mandated by the hegemonic forces. And they draw on a wide variety of influences to do so.

In several of the chapters, the formation of sexuality in youth is a central focus (see Dickey Young, Shipley, Yip, and Boisvert). Youth is seen as a time of impressionable sexuality. For some, this means that youth need to be "protected" from too much information given too soon (see Dickey Young and Shipley). In particular, some religious groups have taken the stance that it is the job of "religion" to police what youth learn about sexuality. For others, the fluidity of youthful sexuality is an important factor in the development of adult sexualities, and the role of religion in providing grist for the development of sexual identity may not always be what religious groups directly intend (see Yip and Boisvert). When youth are allowed to speak for themselves on religion and sexuality, one often hears very different emphases than when youth are spoken about and for.

Embodiment is a key theme in discussions of sexuality and religion. The chapters ask whose bodies count and why. Society provides us with specific understandings of ideal, normative bodies, which are fit, are whole (not "handicapped" in some way), and are dressed and presented in fashionable, heterosexually acceptable ways. Religious groups and traditions often have their own versions of these same norms. Sexual activity involves at least one's own body and often the body of another. Sometimes in religion the sexuality of the body has been seen as problematic, a site for transgression. The chapters in this book, each in its own way, challenge the idea that there is any single normative embodiment. At the same time, they also challenge the idea that the body is of no religious consequence. Religious ideas and actions have had profound effects, both positive and negative, on bodies.

Methods and Theories

The book's authors use a variety of research methods, primarily empirical research and interviews, textual and discourse analysis, and narrative, both personal narratives and those of others. Methodologically, all the authors understand that there is a difference between lived religion – religion embodied in people's everyday lives – and religion as officially presented by religious groups and authorities. The use of a variety of methods allows the book as a whole to highlight a number of different ways of learning about both sexuality and religion.

As noted above, all the authors in this book agree that both religion and sexuality are socially constructed and therefore that our religious and sexual identities are socially constructed through hegemonies, societal forces, and individual decisions. Some of the authors (see Yip, Holtmann, and Nason-Clark) also make explicit that the subjects of their research may not understand their own identities as similarly fluid, and it is also clear that religious and other organizations often approach both religion and sexuality as static "givens" rather than as ever-changing. Further, none of the authors in this volume thinks that the fluidity of either religion or sexuality allows us to avoid thinking about the ethical implications of our theorizing, and several chapters suggest directions in which change might occur (see Jakobsen, Trothen, and Nason-Clark).

Another commonality among the authors is an agreement that religious diversity and sexual diversity are not only empirical facts but also goods to be embraced rather than problems to be solved. Certainly, diversities of any kind might need to be managed for the well-being of individuals and societies, but managing diversity does not mean reducing it to any one manifestation of either sexuality or religion. When identity descriptors beyond religion and sexuality such as race or geographic origin are invoked, they are examined for their role in creating or maintaining certain kinds of normative identities (see Lee).

Beyond the general agreement that identities are not essentialist, the authors employ a wide range of theoretical lenses to allow them to illuminate their own particular subjects, including feminist theory, queer theory, postcolonial theory, and critiques of neoliberalism. Such a variety of methods and theories clearly illustrates that scholars working in this developing field of the study of the intersection of sex and religion are not restricted to just a few approaches to their subject matter.

What Work Is Still to Be Done? What Do We Expect Our Work to Do?

We see this work as a beginning point. Studies of the intersections between sexuality and religion that look beyond religion as regulatory are relatively new. Here, although we explore some of the ways that religion functions to regulate sexuality, we are clear that religion cannot be reduced to regulation. We also agree that religious identities and sexual identities are not two discrete matters that can be separated in creating a personal identity for oneself. Both religion and sexuality take many forms and are embodied in many ways.

We see this book as a contribution to discussions among religious persons and groups, discussions among those of diverse sexualities, discussions that bring religion and sexuality into the same conversation, and discussions concerning public policy-making that see both religion and sexuality as more complex and varied than they often appear to be at first glance.

The desire of the authors in this volume to move beyond tolerance and accommodation begs the question of what we are moving toward. In their chapters, both Janet Jakobsen and Pamela Dickey Young begin articulations of what this might look like. Jakobsen articulates a view of justice wherein diverse participants get to contribute to the formation of the ideal and the practice of justice. Dickey Young, drawing on the work of Lori Beaman, works out some beginning moves toward "deep equality." Deep equality requires that we make space for a wide variety of voices and positions to be both heard and seriously considered. In the context of this volume, such space is made for religious minorities and sexual minorities. Deep equality does not require that one forgo all judgment about various positions, but it does require that the criteria for judgments be clear and transparent. Deep equality requires an expansive capacity for self-critique of the ways that one's own normative assumptions limit the humanity of others. It is crucial to move beyond the idea that we have to decide who is the more discriminated against. Otherwise, it will be difficult to move toward affirmations of human dignity for all.

Issues involving sexuality are often flashpoints for discussions of religious diversity. Non-normative sexuality (however it is defined) is often seen as a problem by religious groups. Those who do not identify with religion often see issues of sexuality within religion as venues for a critique that reduces entire religious traditions to the claim that they oppress women or sexual minorities. Such reductionism does not aid in the understanding of either religious or sexual diversity. We hope that this book helps to move readers beyond such reductionism by exposing the complexity of the relationships between religion and sexuality and by illustrating that to attend to this relationship is to attend not to sweeping themes but to specific venues and instances. Embracing diversity does not mean allowing everything to pass without critique. But it does mean paying more attention to the tendency to construct "others" through overgeneralization. The chapters in this book contribute to resisting such overgeneralization.

References

Beaman, L. 2003. The Myth of Pluralism, Diversity, and Vigor: The Constitutional Privilege of Protestantism in the United States and Canada. *Journal for the Scientific Study of Religion* 42 (3): 311-25.

Contributors

Donald L. Boisvert, a co-investigator on the Religion and Diversity Project, is an associate professor and chair in the Department of Religion, Concordia University, Montreal, where he also teaches in the Sexuality Studies program. In addition to several articles, he is the author of *Out on Holy Ground: Meditations on Gay Men's Spirituality* (2000) and *Sanctity and Male Desire: A Gay Reading of Saints* (2004). He is the co-editor, with Jay Emerson Johnson, of the two-volume collection *Queer Religion* (2012).

Catherine Holtmann has a doctorate in sociology from the University of New Brunswick (UNB), Fredericton. Her research interests lie in the areas of religion and gender, immigrants, and domestic violence. She has worked in a variety of Catholic ministries, as a contract academic instructor at UNB and St. Thomas University in Fredericton, and is active in the Catholic Network for Women's Equality in Canada (http://www.cnwe.org). In addition to serving as a research assistant with the Religion and Violence e-Learning (RAVE) Project (http://www.theraveproject.org), she has helped to develop online teaching resources for the Religion and Diversity Project (http://religionanddiversity.ca).

Janet R. Jakobsen is Ann Whitney Olin Professor of Women's, Gender and Sexuality Studies at Barnard College, Columbia University, where she has also served as dean for Faculty Diversity and Development. She is the author of *Working Alliances and the Politics of Difference: Diversity and*

Feminist Ethics (1998). With Ann Pellegrini, she is co-author of *Love the Sin: Sexual Regulation and the Limits of Religious Tolerance* (2003) and co-editor of *Secularisms* (2008).

Lee Wing Hin has a doctorate from the School of Women's Studies at York University, Toronto. She is interested in how policies and studies on religion, multiculturalism, and immigration have affected Canadian communities of colour and how these communities have, in turn, created or resisted political and social change.

Nancy Nason-Clark is a professor and chair in the Department of Sociology, University of New Brunswick, Fredericton. She received her doctorate from the London School of Economics and Political Science, England, and has been engaged in research and writing on the intersection of religion, gender, culture, and domestic violence for the past twenty-five years. Her books include *The Battered Wife: How Christians Confront Family Violence* (1997), *Refuge from Abuse: Hope and Healing for Abused Christian Women* (co-author, 2004), *No Place for Abuse: Biblical and Practical Resources to Counteract Domestic Violence*, 2nd ed. (co-author, 2010), and *Men Who Batter* (co-author, 2014). For six years, she was editor of *Sociology of Religion: A Quarterly Review,* and she has served as president of the Association for the Sociology of Religion, the Religious Research Association, and Peace and Safety in the Christian Home (PASCH).

Heather Shipley (PhD) is project manager for the Religion and Diversity Project (http://religionanddiversity.ca) and teaches part-time at the University of Ottawa and Carleton University. Her research focuses on the construction, management, and regulation of religion, gender, sexuality, and sexual orientation as identity categories in law, policy, and public discourse. Her publications include "Belief, Not Religion: Youth Negotiations of Religious Identity in Canada," in *Handbook on Child and Youth Studies,* ed. J. Wyn and H. Cahill (co-author, 2014); "Human Rights, Sexuality and Religion: Between Policy and Identity," *Canadian Diversity* 9, 3 (2012): 52-55; and "One of These Things Is Not Like the Other: Regulating Sexual Difference," in *Reasonable Accommodation: Managing Religious Diversity,* ed. L. Beaman (2012).

Tracy J. Trothen is an associate professor at the School of Religion, Queen's University, Kingston, Ontario. She is also a certified Clinical Pastoral Education Supervisor (Canadian Association of Spiritual Care). Trothen is the author of numerous publications, including *Shattering the Illusion: Child Sexual Abuse and Canadian Religious Institutions* (2012). She is co-editor of the forthcoming volume *Religion and Transhumanism: The Unknown Future of Human Enhancement* (Praeger, 2014). Currently she is writing a book on religion, sport, and enhancement technoscience (Mercer University Press, forthcoming).

Andrew Kam-Tuck Yip is a professor of sociology at the University of Nottingham, England. His publications include *Lesbian, Gay and Bisexual Lives over 50* (co-author, 2003), *Queer Spiritual Spaces: Sexuality and Sacred Places* (co-editor, 2010), *Religion, Youth and Sexuality: Selected Key Findings from a Multi-faith Exploration* (co-author, 2011), *The Ashgate Research Companion to Contemporary Religion and Sexuality* (co-editor, 2012), *Religion, Gender and Sexuality in Everyday Life* (co-editor, 2012), and *Religious and Sexual Identities: A Multi-faith Exploration of Young Adults* (co-author 2013).

Pamela Dickey Young is a professor at the School of Religion, Queen's University, Kingston, Ontario. Her research interests concern the intersections of religion, sex, gender, and public policy. Her most recent research project (with Heather Shipley, University of Ottawa) is a study entitled Religion, Gender and Sexuality among Youth in Canada. Her publications include *Religion, Sex and Politics: Christian Churches and Same-Sex Marriage in Canada* (2012); "It's All about Sex: The Opposition of Some Canadian Churches to Gay and Lesbian Marriages," in *Faith Politics and Sexual Diversity in Canada and the United States*, ed. D. Rayside and C. Wilcox (2011); and *Women and Religious Traditions*, 3rd ed. (co-editor, 2014).

Index

abortion, 23-24, 36, 72, 77, 79, 146, 148, 150, 151, 159
accommodation, 7, 60, 108
accountability, 220, 236
activists
    gay/lesbian, 9, 35-36, 74, 136
    Hong Kong Canadians, 69, 81
agency
    individual, 150, 208, 236
    cooperative, 208
    individual choice, 202-3
    making choices, 203, 223, 229
    moral agency, 143, 151, 157
    religious agency, 143, 153
Alberta, 46, 49-51, 52
Alberta Guide to Education, 48
Alberta Human Rights Act, 56
Alberta Human Rights Commission, 46, 48, 49
Alberta School Boards Association, 45
Alberta School Councils' Association, 45
Alberta Teachers' Association, 45, 66
alcoholism: Alcoholics Anonymous (AA), 229

Ammerman, Nancy, 120, 142, 223
Anderson, Rob, 50, 56
androcentric/androcentrism, 143, 147, 149
autonomy, 33, 203
    and consent, 202, 203
    and paternalism, 202

Bannerji, Himani, 78-79
battered
    wife, 225, 229
    woman, 223
Beaman, Lori, 53, 59, 60-61, 243, 245, 248
Benedict XVI (pope), 147, 160n3
Bible/biblical
    gospel, 72, 147, 148
    scripture, 131, 143, 145, 159
Bill 44 (Alberta), 45-46, 48, 55-56, 61, 98
binaries: dichotomies, 112, 144, 194, 209, 210
biopolitics, 31-32
biopower, 30, 32, 143
birth control, 24, 146
Blackett, Lindsay, 46, 48, 51, 56, 64n9

body/bodies, 121, 170, 177, 183, 209
   abused bodies, 225, 235
   embodied/embodiment, 12-13, 166-68, 191-212, 213n1, 243
Boisvert, Donald, 12, 149, 221, 241, 242, 243
Bosco, St. John, 185-87
boundaries, 22, 29, 39, 144, 205, 221, 234, 237
Buddhism/Buddhist, 120

Canadian Charter of Rights and Freedoms, 60, 68
Canadians: Chinese Canadians, 67, 69, 73-79, 83
canonization, 175, 179, 183
Catholic/Catholicism. *See* Roman Catholicism
chasteness/chastity, 176, 178-79, 181-82, 187
child/children, 23-24, 37-38, 47-48, 50-51, 55, 57-58, 62, 101-3, 105, 107, 109, 142, 151-53, 155, 159, 169-70, 176-78, 185, 187, 206, 223-26, 228-29, 235
Christian/Christianity
   Evangelical, 36, 52-54, 56-57, 68-69, 71-77, 80-81 231
   Protestant, 22, 33, 39, 52-53, 57-59, 69, 112, 121, 222, 231
   Roman Catholic. *See* Roman Catholicism
church
   church teachings, 141
   congregation, 36, 73, 156, 222, 225, 228, 230, 232, 233-34, 236
   diocese/diocesan, 142, 145, 149, 156
   ministry, 142, 144, 148, 152, 231 233
   parishioner/parish, 141, 145, 150, 153-59, 230-32
   women-church, 144-45

citizenship, 29, 31, 45-46, 80, 134
College of Alberta School Superintendents, 45
colonial/colonialism, 60-61, 68, 70-71, 73, 79, 81-89
   violence, 81
community, 23-24, 69, 71, 78, 119, 124-27, 149, 155-58, 172, 222, 224-25, 228, 230-36
   communities of faith, 220, 223
conservative, 22, 24, 28, 35, 46, 50-52, 55-59, 68-70, 83, 121, 144-45, 222, 231
contraception, 24, 146
control, 21, 30-36, 46, 58, 80, 85, 121-22, 146, 171, 175, 182, 184, 186-87, 211, 221, 224, 236, 243,
criminal justice system, 222
   crime, 148
   law enforcement, 226
curriculum, 46, 48, 54, 97-113

desire, 35-39, 47, 78, 97, 121-24, 135, 170-80, 184-85, 191-92, 206-7, 211, 221
Desiring Change project, 35-37
difference, 233
dignity, 62, 141, 146-47, 245
discourse, 21, 34, 56, 68, 70-74, 17, 83-86, 105, 108-13, 119, 122, 125, 129-31, 134, 143, 170, 182, 185, 187
   public discourse, 29, 31-32, 70, 97, 99-101, 107, 110, 113, 134, 221
diversity
   and embodiment, 192-93, 197-200, 204, 206, 208-11
   of leadership, 145
   religious, 22, 25, 39, 59-60, 171
   sexual, 21-22, 59-60, 66, 98, 105-7, 110-11
doctrine, 59, 101, 111, 145-46
   Papal encyclical, 146

Duggan, Lisa, 29, 38, 70, 100, 110

Economic and Social Research Council (UK), 137
economic(s), 23-25, 29, 31, 35-39, 82, 143, 147, 151, 158-59, 202, 224
  economic institutions, 147
  poor, 29, 142-43, 151, 186
  poverty, 23, 35, 72, 81-82, 158-59
education
  faith-based, 49, 226
  seminary students, 233-34
  sex education, 24, 54, 97-113
  training, 200, 206, 226, 231, 234
enhancement (of bodies), 192-212
  doping, 197, 199, 200
epistemology, 194
  categories, 132, 136, 194
equality, 25, 39, 80, 101, 119, 134, 209
  deep equality, 60-62
Equality Act (UK, 2010), 134
essentialisms, 100, 101, 105; essential nature, 148
esteem: self-esteem, 224
ethics
  ethical problem, 152
  moral, 29-32, 36, 39, 72-77
  sexual, 36, 39, 130, 135, 147
  theological ethic, 194
ethnic minority, 69, 72
Evangelical(s). *See* Christian/Christianity
experience: personal, 136, 150, 171, 231

fairness, 38, 136, 152, 200, 203, 205
  unfair, 198, 200, 204, 205
faith: religious, 83, 123, 125, 127-33, 145, 154-56, 158, 180, 211, 220, 222-27, 231, 233, 236

family/families, 24, 28, 30, 34, 36, 37, 39, 50-51, 62, 79, 105, 113, 141, 159, 222-36
father(s)/fatherhood, 23, 24, 38
feminism, 191
  feminist movement, 144, 232
  feminist theology, 158
forgiveness, 181, 224
Foucault, Michel, 22, 30, 99, 122, 191, 193
Francis, Pope, 147, 175
freedom
  religious freedom/freedom of religion, 21, 26, 60, 73, 79, 101
  sexual freedom, 32, 33, 143

gay, 26, 28, 35, 50-51, 54, 73, 98, 100, 120, 123, 126, 143, 187, 192
gender, 22-25, 29, 35-36, 101, 122, 129-31, 188, 191, 198, 201, 221-22, 236
  categories, 205, 213n5
  gendered approach, 146
  identity, 100, 102, 104-5, 109, 111-13, 134, 179
genetics, 197-201
  genetic advantages, 197
  genetic anomalies, 201
  germ-line genetic modification, 197, 213n6
  Repoxygen, 197, 198, 203
God, 33, 48, 71-74, 80-83, 109, 122, 130, 132-33, 135-36, 142, 151, 152, 155, 224, 225, 227-28, 236
Goretti, St. Maria, 179-85, 188
guilt(y), 124, 132, 150, 154, 171, 177, 198, 224

hagiography, 177
Hancock, Dave, 48
healing, 127, 152, 220, 223, 225, 234, 236
hegemony, 25, 59-60, 184-85, 243

heteronormative/heteronormativity, 34, 56, 59, 112, 122, 125, 130-31, 136, 143
heterosexual/heterosexuality, 51-57, 62, 100, 103, 119-30, 133, 135, 137*n*10, 170, 191-94, 242-43
hierarchy, 26, 84, 86, 145-46, 156, 159
Holtmann, Cathy, 145, 148-49, 155, 157, 194, 196, 203, 221, 234, 241, 242, 244
home, 47, 51, 101, 109, 156, 185-86, 223-26, 228, 230
homogeneity, 78
homophobia/homophobic, 50, 72, 134
homosexuality, 57, 68, 72-74, 76, 79, 81, 111, 121
Hong Kong Canadian, 35, 67-87
hope, 131, 159, 206-12, 220
human rights, 38, 45-51, 56, 73, 98, 106, 134-35
humiliation, 221
Hunt, Stephen, 121

iconography, 177, 187
identity
    multiple identities, 143
    norms, 99
    religious identity, 98, 110, 113, 125, 142, 171, 221, 236
    sexual identity, 60, 100, 102, 106, 109-11, 180, 243
immigrants, 22, 27, 28, 39, 69, 72-79, 81-83, 87, 108
integration, 119-21, 127, 130-31, 133-34
    of beliefs, 127, 133
    cultural integration, 88*n*8
Islam: Muslim, 105, 108, 120, 124-29, 131
Islamophobia, 126

Jakobsen, Janet, 26-28, 33, 35, 60, 71, 99, 111-13, 134, 143, 203, 211

John Paul II (pope), 147, 175, 183
Jubilee Centre for Christian Social Action (JCCSA), 77
Judaism/Jewish, 22, 27, 123
justice
    economic justice, 35, 37
    inequalities, 146, 147
    social action, 77, 144, 146, 150, 155, 159
    social justice, 135-36, 142, 145-46, 148-49, 154, 157, 236

Lee, Wing Hin, 67-92
lesbian, 26, 35, 50, 54, 68, 98, 100, 120, 122-23, 130, 131, 143
lesbian, gay, bisexual (LGB), 120, 125-27, 130-33, 135-36
liberal/liberalism, 24, 27-28, 39, 55, 69, 202
    liberal democracy, 202
liminal/liminality, 109, 176, 182
logos schools, 47, *63n3*

marriage, 30, 33, 5, 39, 53, 54, 60, 69, 125, 128, 130, 148, 154
    divorce, 79, 141, 153-54, 232
    reform, 73, 84
    same-sex, 57, 67-69, 71-72, 74-78, 81, 87
    traditional, 67-68
martyr/martyrdom, 172, 179-80, 183-84
McGuinty, Dalton (Ontario), 99, 102, 106-7, 109, 112
McGuire, Meredith, 161, 120, 144, 223
media, 53, 69, 73, 97, 99-101, 105-7, 110, 169, 194, 207
memory, 172-74
men, 23, 38, 75, 123, 147, 152, 182, 184, 187, 191-92, 220, 222
minorities
    religious, 61, 108, 110

sexual, 57, 59, 110, 131, 242
moral panic(s), 29-30, 105-6, 242
Morosini, Blessed Pierina, 183
mothers/motherhood, 29, 38, 147, 148, 157
multiculturalism, 45, 49, 55, 60-61, 67-68, 70-73, 76-80, 83, 108
   Multiculturalism Act (Canada, 1971), 49

narrative, 39, 70-71, 78, 83-86, 110-12, 130, 171-72, 174, 177-78, 221, 234-36, 244
Nason-Clark, Nancy, 143, 249, 154, 172, 194, 220, 222, 230-31, 242, 244
nationalism, 70-71, 74, 80
natural, 110, 197, 200-1, 209
   and artificial, 209
normal, 29, 50, 51, 56, 101, 110, 127, 136, 190, 200-2, 209
nuns, 142, 149, 152, 171, 176, 181

Obama, Barack, 22-25
Office of Faith-Based and Neighborhood Partnerships, 22-25
oppression, 129, 131, 135-36, 143, 145, 147, 154

panoptic gaze, 122
patriarchy/patriarchal, 39, 143, 147, 156, 170, 182, 183
pedagogy, 171, 173, 176, 177, 181, 188
Pellegrini, Ann, 26-27, 32, 60, 99, 111-13
pluralism, 21, 22, 57, 59-61, 119-20
politics/political, 35, 39, 51, 55-56, 68-70, 72, 74-85, 111,112, 120, 129, 132-36
   political correctness, 73, 80
   sexual politics, 22, 28-30, 36, 37, 135
postmodernism, 193-94

power, 30-32, 74, 83, 85, 98-99, 122, 143, 144, 147, 176, 182-85, 203
   power dynamics, 147
   social power, 147
   submission, 232
prayer, 197-98, 225
pregnancy, 23, 102, 104, 141
priesthood, 180
private, 37-38, 46, 51-52, 62-63, 183, 185
   private sphere, 36, 62, 147, 221
   public and private, 47, 62
prosthetics, 190, 197
Protestant(s)/Protestantism. *See* Christian/Christianity
Puar, Jasbir, 31, 70
purity, 170, 176, 180-85, 187, 188, 221

queer/queers, 21, 24, 26, 28-29, 34, 36-39, 70, 100, 110, 113, 126, 143, 174, 196, 242, 244
queer theory, 24, 100, 113
Queers for Economic Justice, 35, 37

race/racism, 29, 38-39, 50, 61, 70, 73, 76, 79-80, 83, 130, 143, 191, 198-99, 244
referrals, 231-32, 234
   fear of making, 230
relationship, 34, 36, 38-39, 57, 103-4, 111-12, 120, 123, 124-25, 128-32, 143-44, 152-54, 226-27, 231-32
   relationship counselling, 231
religion/religious
   religiosity, 22, 62, 125, 144-45, 242
   religious convictions, 55, 143, 220, 224
   religious leaders/pastors/clergy, 25, 73, 76, 145, 154, 159, 181, 222, 230-32, 236
   secular religion, 192, 194, 196, 209-11

Religion, Youth and Sexuality: A Multi-Faith Exploration (UK), 137*nn*1-2
remorse, 234
reproduction, 86, 98
    reproductive choice, 142-43, 146, 148-49, 152-53
research
    focus groups, 149, 153, 222, 233
    interviews, 149, 153, 222, 231, 244
    qualitative, 123, 127, 145, 222
    quantitative, 127, 222
resilience, 81, 87, 136
resistance, 115*n*15, 136, 156, 159, 223
resources
    cultural, 144
    spiritual, 149, 221
Roman Catholicism, 53, 142, 155, 173-74, 177, 179
    Canadian Catholic Church, 159
    Catholic social teachings, 142, 146-47, 149-54, 156, 158
    religious orders, 144, 149, 151, 155, 186
    Vatican Council, 142, 146, 155

safety, 26, 199, 224-25, 229-30, 234-35
    fear, 51, 72, 170, 225, 229-30, 233-34
    personal safety, 230
saint/saints, 171-89
Savio, St. Dominic, 179-80, 185-86
Scarborough Chinese Baptist Church Fellowship, 73
school(s), 46-48, 50-55, 58, 59, 61-63, 84, 105, 181, 187
secular/secularism, 22-23, 25, 27-28, 32-35, 39, 53-54, 59, 73, 81, 110-12, 119, 125, 129, 133-35, 143-44, 149, 150, 192, 225, 231-37
    sacred/secular dichotomy, 144
sex/sexual/sexuality
    heteronormative, 112, 125, 131, 145

orientation, 45, 48-62, 100, 102, 105, 110-13, 125, 134-35
    sexual desire, 122, 128, 174, 178, 191
    sexual expression, 221
    sexual panic, 70
    sexual practice, 191, 211
    women's sexuality, 141, 146, 149, 160*n*3, 160*n*7
sex education curriculum (Ontario), 97-113
sexism, 147
sexual orientation: lesbian/gay/queer/heterosexual/homosexual/intersexed, 45, 48, 49, 50-62, 100-2, 105, 109-13, 125, 134-35, 143
shame, 124, 132, 133, 177
Sheldon Chumir Foundation for Ethics in Leadership, 46
Shipley, Heather, 221, 234, 243
silence: culture of, 221, 234, 243
social construction, 144, 191, 242
social movements, 36, 136
    religious, 71
spatial analysis, 98, 107
spirit
    sacred, 121, 143-44, 170, 176, 184-85, 195-96, 209, 220, 232, 235
    spiritual issues, 225
    spirituality, 81, 121, 132, 175, 179, 209
    strong in, 235
sport
    athlete(s), 190, 192, 194, 196-206, 210, 211-12
    Olympics, 190-91, 194, 196, 201, 204-5, 207, 209-10
    Paralympics, 190, 204, 209
Stelmach, Ed, 47, 48
suffering, 177
Supreme Court of Canada, 54, 68
survivors, 152, 220-22, 225, 230

techno-science, 192, 193, 197, 199, 203, 205-8, 210-12
theology/theological, 83, 120, 133, 144-47, 152, 155, 158, 184, 188, 191-99, 203, 205-8
therapy
  counsellors, 231
  pastoral care, 146, 151
  psychologists, 230
  therapeutic, 151, 222, 235
  therapists, 230
tolerance, 26-28, 34, 36, 54, 60, 72, 80, 112, 241, 242, 245, 248
Toronto Chinese Evangelical Ministerial (TCEMF), 73, 76, 77, 89n10
tradition, 24, 28, 36-37, 78, 155, 157, 159, 178
transcendence, 191, 192, 195-96
  and immanence, 196
transformation, 130-33
transgender(ed), 24, 26, 37
transgression, 130, 243
Trothen, Tracy, 192, 195, 197, 200, 202, 210
Tse, Dominic (Pastor), 76-79, 82

United Kingdom, 40n3, 119-20, 134, 208, 242-43
United States, 21, 22, 26-29, 32-33, 36, 38-39, 53, 60, 199, 208, 236, 243

values
  Christian, 27, 59
  family, 24, 25, 39
  liberal, 28
  secular, 28
victims, 84, 142-43, 151-52, 155, 221, 230, 232-33
violence
  abuse, 84, 141, 143, 147, 151-59, 176, 188, 220-23, 225-26, 229-37
  date rape, 142, 148, 150, 151, 159, 180-82, 184, 150
  domestic, 141, 142, 148, 153-54, 158-59, 220-26, 229-36, 237n5
  institutionalized violence, 147
  intimate partner violence, 141, 142, 147
  name calling, 221
  rape/sexual assault/sexual violence, 29, 151, 182
  spousal violence, 147, 148
  violence against women, 148, 153
virgin/virginity/virginal, 169, 176, 178, 180-84, 187
virtue/virtuous, 175-78, 185, 187-88, 221
vulnerable, 51, 223, 226

Weber, Max, 33
World War II, 75, 82-83

Yip, Andrew Kam-Tuck, 100, 121, 127, 130-33
Young, Pamela Dickey, 100, 196
youth/young, 101-3, 111, 119, 120, 121, 155, 157, 159, 169-74, 176-82, 184-88, 226, 243

Printed and bound in Canada by Friesens

Set in Univers and Minion by Artegraphica Design Co. Ltd.

Copy editor: Robert Lewis

Proofreader: Helen Godolphin